Adolescent Schizophrenia

ADOLESCENT SCHIZOPHRENIA

JAMES T. NILLINGHOUSE
AND
ROBERT P. TROTMAN
EDITORS

Nova Biomedical Books
New York

For permission to use material from this book please contact us:
Telephone 631-231-7269; Fax 631-231-8175
Web Site: http://www.novapublishers.com

Library of Congress Cataloging-in-Publication Data

Adolescent schizophrenia / editors, James T. Nillinghouse and Robert P. Trotman.

p. ; cm.

Includes bibliographical references and index.

ISBN 978-1-60692-370-2 (hardcover)

1. Schizophrenia in adolescence. I. Nillinghouse, James T. II. Trotman, Robert P.

[DNLM: 1. Schizophrenia--physiopathology. 2. Adolescent. 3. Schizophrenia--therapy. WM 203 A239 2009]

RJ506.S3A36 2009

616.89'800835--dc22

2008050988

Published by Nova Science Publishers, Inc. ✣ New York

Contents

Preface

Schizophrenia is a chronic disorder that impacts a broad range of a person's social and developmental functioning. Until the recent past, most of the research done on schizophrenia did not include children or adolescents who suffer from the disorder.

During adolescence, important changes take place in brain development. These changes make adolescence a period of both vulnerability and opportunity. Emergence of psychosis and schizophrenia may be associated with abnormal brain development during adolescence. This book discusses the findings of studies that focus on abnormal brain development during the premorbid period of psychosis and schizophrenia.

Cognitive neuroscience constructs of visuospatial memory and working memory are associated with adult- and adolescent-onset schizophrenia. This book reviews the existing literature on the topic and explores the nature of and association between visuospatial memory in adolescent onset schizophrenia.

The prevalence of psychotic symptoms in the general population, particularly in children and adolescents, is also explored. The significance of psychotic symptoms in relation to psychiatric disorders, such as depression and anxiety, and its relation to social factors, such as childhood abuse is examined.

To deal with schizophrenic young patients in a hospital, psychoanalytical psychotherapeutic "teamwork" is reviewed. The transference relation between patient and therapist, and what it entails, is also discussed.

Chapter I - During adolescence, important changes take place in the brain development. These changes make adolescence a period of both vulnerability and opportunity. Emergence of psychosis and schizophrenia may be associated with abnormal brain development during adolescence. In this chapter, first, we describe findings of structural and functional MRI studies related to some of the deviant behaviors during adolescence, in the context of risks and opportunities associated with brain development in this period. Second, we focus on findings of studies of abnormal brain development during the premorbid period of psychosis in general, and of szhizophrenia, in particular.

Chapter II - This chapter investigates the nature of and association between visuospatial memory, and, separately, visuospatial working memory in adolescent onset schizophrenia. The data presented suggest that both the visuospatial memory and working memory performance of the adolescent-onset schizophrenia group are impaired compared to the healthy control group. Further, the type and magnitude of the deficits are similar to those reported in the adult-onset schizophrenia patients suggesting these deficits are developmental stage independent. The import of these findings is examined within the context of emerging neurobiological models of progressive parietal-temporal-frontal linked neural network dysfunction in schizophrenia, whether of adolescent- or adult-onset. Also, the implications of these findings for the current aetiological understanding of schizophrenia and the current assessment and treatment approaches are discussed.

Chapter III - Recent studies suggest that psychosis exists along a continuum in the general population, rather than as an all-or-none phenomenon. This is supported by the finding that the prevalence of psychotic symptoms in the general population far exceeds the prevalence of psychotic disorders. Only 1% of the overall population will develop schizophrenia during their lifetime whereas international epidemiological research suggests that between 5% and 38% of the adult general population may experience at least one psychotic symptom in their lives, with rates of 2.1% to 58.9 % reported for child and adolescent populations. The significance of psychotic symptoms in children and adolescents is not as yet fully established: they have been found to be associated with a variety of psychiatric disorders in this age group, in particular depression and anxiety, and social factors including childhood abuse. There is emerging evidence that psychotic symptoms in childhood and adolescence may be risk markers for psychotic illness in adulthood. Poulton et al (1999) [1] found that self-reported psychotic symptoms at age 11 years predicted a very high risk of a schizophrenia spectrum disorder at age 26 years. Therefore, adolescents who report psychotic symptoms could be conceptualised as a 'high risk' group for schizophrenia. This paradigm may prove valuable in exploring early risk factors for psychosis-vulnerability and in predicting psychotic outcomes.

Chapter IV - Psychoanalytical psychotherapeutic "teamwork" may be recommended for dealing with this particular kind of mental pathology characterized by schizophrenic symptoms in young patients. In such cases, the degree of alienation is such that repetition is usually induced in other people (the therapists), filling in for fantasy construction that seems then to be lacking in the patient's psyche. A case like that of "Angel" can give some idea of this phenomenon, wherein several caregivers have to harbor fragmented and incompatible elements of the case's particular history, which are in need of more mental representation. Any subjective restitution and appropriation of these elements by the patient would require a sort of detour (often a trying one!) by way of the psychical space of caregivers whose initial task will be to "work it through" among themselves.

Chapter V - Treatment of psychiatric disorders is hampered by the fact that their causes are poorly understood. Our ignorance is even deeper when it comes to aggressive behavior in psychiatric patients. Clearly, without better understanding of underlying neuropsychobiology of aggression we cannot improve the existing treatments. This chapter therefore first reviews neurobiological and psychosocial factors affecting aggression in schizophrenia, and then proceeds to discuss their implications for treatment. Finally, the current state of the psychopharmacology of aggression in schizophrenia is briefly reviewed.

Chapter VI - Background

Body image aberration in schizophrenia was earlier conceived as delusional and hallucinatory symptoms. However, perceptions of schizophrenia have changed dramatically, especially with the concept of negative symptoms in the 1980s and in the 1990s, to include the neurocognitive aspects of schizophrenia. Deviations in schizophrenics' body image from the standard underlying various behaviors or allegations concerning the body should be now refocused. In this chapter, using the Body Image Questionnaire (BIQ), comprised of three hypothetical components, anatomical, functional and psychological, attempts were made to resolve some primary questions. They were (1) whether or not there is any related clinical characteristics to schizophrenic body image abberation, (2) whether there are aberrant components of body image specific to schizophrenia, (3) whether or not there is unique link between depression and body image in schizophrenia.

Methods

In study 1, correlations between body image assessed by the BIQ and clinical characteristics as positive and negative symptoms assessed by SAPS and SANS, insight assessed by SAI, and daily dose of conventional antipsychotic drugs were examined. In study 2, three components of body image, that is, anatomical, functional and psychological, were compared between schizophrenic and non-schizophrenic groups. In study 3, the correlation between depression assessed by SDS and body image assessed by the BIQ was examined. In these studies, 93 chronic schizophrenics, 177 normal adults, and 43 patients with anxiety disorders according to DSM-IV criteria, were examined. In studies 4-5, the additional finding of Rorschach percepts concerning body image in schizophrenia was reported.

Results

Schizophrenics' body image aberration proved to be independent of symptoms and medication. It was also shown that the aberration proved to be limited to functional imageries, and that the anatomical component remained intact. As to depression, a specific link of body image, especially with functional imageries, with the depression characteristic to schizophrenia was found.

Conclusion

All these results showed that body image aberration in schizophrenics is not the result of symptoms or effects of conventional neuroleptic medications, but they are germane to schizophrenia, which is comprised of aberration mainly in functional body imageries. This body image deviation proved to be linked to some serious depressive signs and symptoms in schizophrenia. The subsidiary findings, that is, the Rorschach percepts as a mass of flesh quite often seen in schizophrenia, are congruent with the main findings that schizophrenic patients showed an anticipation of becoming unmovable.

Chapter VII - There is a well-documented link between schizophrenia and antisocial behavior. For example, studies of violent offenders worldwide find a significantly elevated prevalence of schizophrenia and spectrum disorder diagnoses (Gosden, Kramp, Gabrielsen, and Sestoft, 2003; Arseneault, Moffitt, Caspi, Taylor, and Silva, 2000). Conversely, studies of patient populations reveal higher rates of antisocial behavior. In an investigation of a large

Danish birth cohort in their forties, proportionately more of the men and women who developed schizophrenia were convicted of non-violent and violent crimes (Brennan, Mednick, and Hodgins, 2000). Similar results were obtained in investigations of population cohorts in Australia (Mullen, Burgess, Wallace, Palmer, and Ruschena, 2000), Israel (Stueve and Link, 1997), and New Zealand (Arseneault et al., 2000).

Investigations into the specific links between symptoms and antisocial behavior suggest that the severity of positive symptoms is the strongest predictor of aggressive and violent behavior. Further, some findings indicate that individuals at risk for developing schizophrenia and spectrum disorders are more likely to manifest antisocial behaviors. The link between premorbid antisocial behavior and psychosis has been examined in both retrospective and prospective longitudinal studies. In a retrospective study of childhood-onset schizophrenia, Schaeffer and Ross (2002) found a high proportion of parents reporting oppositional behavior, violence, aggression, temper tantrums, and rages as premorbid signs in their children. Similarly, Arsenault et al. (2000) found that individuals with schizophrenia-spectrum disorders were more likely to have a childhood history of conduct disorder.

Chapter VIII - Risk factors for mortality and morbidity are divisible into three categories: those present before conception, others occurring postpartum and finally, those that operate in the interval between conception and birth. Until comparatively recently, this last period received limited attention in epidemiological research on psychiatric and (to a lesser degree) other disorders first emerging beyond the childhood years. One notable exception is the early and sustained interest in possible prenatal viral etiology of schizophrenia. Nonetheless, the operation of genetic factors, present at conception, and of macro and micro-level environmental factors, in the postnatal period were the primary focus of attention.

Research and Review Studies

In: Adolescent Schizophrenia
Editors: J. T. Nillinghouse and R. P. Trotman
ISBN: 978-1-60692-370-2

Chapter I

Adolescent Brain Development, Behavior, Premorbid Psychosis and Risk for Schizophrenia: A Review of Structural and Functional MRI Studies

Ozgur Oner*
Ankara Diskapi Children's Hospital, Child Psychiatry Department, Ankara, Turkey
NIMH Fogarty International Center Mental Health and Developmental Disabilities (MHDD) Program, Children's Hospital, Boston, USA
Haluk Ozbay
Yildirim Bayazit Hospital Psychiatry Department, Ankara, Turkey
Kerim M. Munir†
Children's Hospital Boston, Harvard Medical School, Division of General Pediatrics and Department of Psychiatry, Boston, USA

Abstract

During adolescence, important changes take place in the brain development. These changes make adolescence a period of both vulnerability and opportunity. Emergence of psychosis and schizophrenia may be associated with abnormal brain development during adolescence. In this chapter, first, we describe findings of structural and functional MRI

* Correspondence concerning this article should be addressed to: Ozgur Oner, M.D., Child Psychiatry Service, Ankara Diskapi Children's Hospital, Advanced in Country Fellow, NIMH Fogarty International Center Mental Health and Developmental Disabilities (MHDD) Program, Children's Hospital, Boston, USA. E-mail: ozz_oner@yahoo.com

† Kerim M Munir, M.D., M.P.H., D.Sc., Children's Hospital Boston, Harvard Medical School, Division of General Pediatrics and Department of Psychiatry, Boston, USA. Tel: 617-818-1853; Fax: 617 730-0049; E-mail: kerim.munir@childrens.harvard.edu

studies related to some of the deviant behaviors during adolescence, in the context of risks and opportunities associated with brain development in this period. Second, we focus on findings of studies of abnormal brain development during the premorbid period of psychosis in general, and of szhizophrenia, in particular.

Introduction

Adolescence is not a simple transiton period from child to adult years, but a time of great maturational change during which important foundations of adult behaviors and emotions are shaped. According to Ronald Dahl, the period of adolescence also signifies a "health paradox" with increases in both physical and cognitive capacities but also associated with rises in morbidity and mortality, related to misjudgments in decision making under stressful and emotion-laden conditions (Dahl, 2004). Many of the stresses especially facing the high-risk youth in concert with ensuing problems their problems in reasoning set the stage for studies examining the neurobiological underpinnings of adolescent behaviors and emotions. For example, novelty seeking, one of the most typical behavioral patterns of adolescence, that helps adolescents to gain independence from their parents, may also lead to increased mortality and morbidity due to the inability of adolescents to calculate risks associated with their immature prefrontal-limbic system network (Kelley et al., 2004).

With respect to studies of brain development during premorbid states, investigating similarities and differences between brain development in normal adolescence and pathological processes during the prodromal phase of psychosis, or schizophrenia, may also yield a better understanding of these serious conditions. Schizophrenia is particularly associated with impaired reality testing, characterised by delusions, hallucinations, and disorganised behaviors. It has been well documented that the prevalence of schizophrenia begins to increase during adolescence. Numerous studies have investigated the behavioral, cognitive, and neurobiological properties during the premorbid period of schizophrenia, which typically includes the adolescents and young adults.

In this chapter, we discuss two lines of complementary research involving the use of structural and functional magnetic resonance imaging (MRI) studies to understand the changes in brain development, and the association of these changes with adolescent behaviors and emotions. First, we describe findings of structural and functional MRI studies related to some of the deviant behaviors during adolescence, in the context of risks and opportunities associated with brain development in this period. Second, we focus on findings of studies of abnormal brain development during the premorbid period of psychosis in general, and of szhizophrenia, in particular.

Brain Development during Adolescence

Sisk and Foster (2004) distinguishes between adolescence and puberty, the former referring to "the maturation of adult social and cognitive behaviors" while latter signalling the "activation of the hypothalamic-pituatry-gonadal axis that culminates in gonadal maturation." The change of behaviors, emotions and cognitions to achieve adult social roles during adolescence is thus clearly related to the social environment. In Western countries the onset of puberty is getting earlier while the assumption of adult roles getting later, so that adolescence may be as long as a decade. In traditional communities the onset of adult roles is considerably earlier and adolescence may merely be as long as 2 to 4 years (Dahl, 2004). It needs to be underscored at the outset therefore, that both the social environment and cultural context needs to be accounted for whenever commenting on the effect of neurobiological factors on behaviors and emotions.

Despite such limitations, the structural and functional magnetic resonance imaging (MRI) techniques can provide invaluable data on the brain development during adolescence. To date, there have been two major types of study designs. Cross-sectional case-comparison studies generally have collected data at one point in time and compared differen individuals in various age groups, while longitudinal studies have followed the same individuals over time. The latter studies have been particularly useful since it has been shown that individual variability may be more prominent than developmental variability (Caviness et al., 1996).

Total brain volume peaks at almost 15 years of age and male brains are 9% bigger than female brains (Giedd et al., 1999). However, inter-individual variability is very high even in normal populations and 50% difference of absolute brain volumes has been reported (Lenroot and Giedd, 2006). Different cortical gray matter volume peaks are observed in various brain regions. Peak frontal and parietal gray matter volumes are reached in 11.0 and 10.0 years in girls and 12.1 and 12.0 years in boys, respectively, while temporal gray matter reaches maximum in 16.7 years in girls and 16.2 years in boys (Giedd et al., 1999). After these peaks, gray matter declines until early adulthood. Another study reported that in the dorsal prefrontal cortex post-pubertal increase in white matter was inversely correlated with decreases in gray matter (Sowell et al., 2001). Caudate nucleus gray matter peaks earlier (7.5 years in girls and 10.0 years in boys) (Giedd et al., 1999) and progressive volume loss is reported particularly in the caudate nucleus (Toga et al., 2006). The gray matter volume changes may be related with gender; it is reported that amygdala and hippocampus volumes increases with age only in males and females, respectively (Giedd et al., 1996), however, there are contradictory findings considering the effect of gender. Gogtay and associates showed that cerebral regions which are phylogenetically older and associated with primary functions mature earlier than phylogenetically newer cerebral association areas (2004). This suggests that the adolescence is a period when previously achieved primary functions are integrated to reach a more effective cerebral function.

Sowell and associates (2004) investigated the change of cortical thickness with age in a longitudinal sample. They reported that cortical thickness decreases with age in the dorsal prefrontal and parietal regions and increased in language related areas of temporal and frontal cortex, suggesting that the changes were related to changing language abilities with age. In the same sample the authors found that greater change of cortical thickness in left dorsal frontal and left parietal cortex was associated with better performance in a general intelligence test. In another study, subjects with higher IQ have shown to experience greater changes in cortical thickness (Shaw et al., 2006). Environmental factors, like training, also effect cortical thickness (Draganski et al., 2004). Recently, it has been shown that heritability of cortical thickness is highest in the brain regions like dorsal frontal, orbitofrontal and temporal cortices, that are associated with higher cognitive functions (Lenroot et al., 2007). These researchers also reported that the heritability of cortical thickness of various brain regions is related to age: heritability of cortical thickness of the philogenetically older brain regions being higher during childhood while heritability of newer cortical regions is higher during adolescence, suggesting a complex relationship between genetic and environmental factors and brain development.

Developmental trajectories of gray and white matter are different. White matter volume increases with age almost linearly during adolescence (Sowell et al., 1999, 2001, 2003, Giedd et al., 1999). In addition, the change of white matter with age is similar in different cerebral regions, like frontal, temporal and parietal cortex (Lenroot and Giedd, 2006). There is a recognizable pattern of myelination with proximal, sensory and projection pathways myelinated before distal, motor and association pathways (Volpe, 2000). Myelination leads to increased intregration of different brain regions and the executive control of the frontal cortex by increasing transmission speed (Luna and Sweeney, 2004). Myelination continues into adolescence and young adulthood in the frontal cortex, suggesting accelarated transmission (Yakovlev and Lecours, 1967, Benes et al., 1994). It must also be kept in mind that brain changes continue well after adolescence, and that white matter increases until 60 years of age (Sowell et al., 2003). More recent studies have showed that dorsal cortex is less myelinated than ventral cortex in its most mature state and that the cortical maturation might in fact occur from a rostral-lateral-ventral pole to a dorsal-medial-caudal pole (Toga et al., 2006, Gogtay et al., 2004), suggesting that the maturation of white matter may be more complex.

Synaptogenesis, the process of increasing synapses, in the prefrontal cortex is very prominent during puberty, followed by synaptic pruning, the process of synaptic elimination, which is prominent during adolescence (Huttenlocher, 1979, Bourgeois et al., 1994). Again, it must be remembered that puberty and adolescence are not identical. Synaptic pruning is an activity-dependent process and, therefore, associated with experience. Pruning may be necessary for more efficient use of cerebal resources and increase in signal to noise ratio. Synaptic pruning includes glutamergic inputs to the prefrontal cortex in particular (Huttenlocher, 1984), while the dopaminergic and sertonergic inputs peak during adolescence (Crews et al., 2007), with later substantial declines. GABAergic interneurons do not change significantly during adolescence, suggesting that experience induced synaptic pruning particularly effects excitatory synapses (Spessot et al., 2004). Thus, pruning does not seem to effect every neorutranmitter system the same way. Synaptic pruning is also seen in amygdala, hippocampus and hypothalamus (Crews et al., 2007). The pubertal increase in gray matter in various cortical regions, and the following decrease until young adulthood, may reflect synaptogesis and synaptic pruning processes, respectively (Giedd et al., 1999). Interestingly, the executive functions performance is *worse* in 11-12 years of age than younger children, suggesting that the increased synpatogenesis during the onset of puberty leads to higher signal-to-noise ratio and worse performance (McGivern et al., 2002). It is also speculated that, similar to the development of the sensory system during early development, the synaptogenesis during puberty may render the brain more sensitive to "experiential inputs" (Blakemore and Choudhury, 2006). Interestingly, the brain regions that mature latest are more susceptible to degenerative diseases like Alzheimer's disease (Toga et al., 2006, Mesulam, 2000). This also suggests that plasticity may be associated with both opportunities and vulnerabilities. On the other hand, a very recent study reported that increased activation in prefrontal and parietal cortex in adults might be due to the increased strength of connectivity between cerebral regions (but not within regions) and that synaptic pruning and myelination are less important (Edin et al., 2007).

Functional neuroimaging studies have the potential to investigate the association of cognitive development with cerebral maturation more directly. The functional MRI studies have shown that cerebral activation changes during various tasks with development. However, the direction of the change is not very clear. Some studies showed that, when combined with worse task performance, high activation in cerebral regions indicates inefficient use of resources (Gaillard et al., 2000). In a study prefrontal activation is found to be increasing with age during Stroop task (Adleman et al., 2002). On the other hand, in another study in which the performance is matched between children and adults, the researchers reported lower prefrontal cortex activation during response inhibition and interference control tasks (Bunge et al., 2002). Another study found that when the performance was segregated from activation, children failed to activate dorsal prefrontal cortex during a single-word processing task as adults (Schlaggar et al., 2002). Similarly, broader activation during cognitive tasks, together with worse performance, points to a less specific activation pattern. With maturation smaller, and more focal regions are activated to perform a similar task (Casey et al., 1997, Durston et al., 2006). This is also reflected in the correlation of cerebral activation with cognitive performance; with maturation the brain regions which are not correlated with task performance are activated less. This suggestion may also be valid for processing of emotional stimuli. Emotional intelligence, the capacity to cope during demanding conditions, is shown to be negatively related to the activity of the limbic system, suggesting more efficient use of the limbic and paralimbic system of high performing individuals (Killgore and Yurgelun-Todd, 2007). It has also been suggested that children might be using compensatory brain regions which are not used in adults during specific tasks (Bunge and Wright, 2007). The activation shifts from subcortical structures to cortical ones during maturation, together with increased connectivity in frontal-subcortical circuits (reviewed in Durston and Casey, 2006).

Another point of interest is performance of adolescents in "hot" vs "cold" situations. Here, "hot" refers to conditions that include or associated with "heightened" emotional states, distraction or competition (Luna and Sweeney, 2004). In rats, it is shown that during the period that corresponds to adolescence in humans, the connectivity between amygdala and prefrontal cortex increases (Cunningham et al., 2002). This is important to suggest that during adolescence the prefrontal (executive) control of the limbic system is not mature. Functional neuroimaging studies also hint on the risk-taking behavior during adolescence. One study reported that the adolescents show less activation in right amygdala and ventral striatum during a task on reward directed behavior when compared to young adults. Authors commented that adolescents may take more risky behaviors to compensate for the lower activation in the neural systems related to motivation (Bjork et al., 2004). Motivation and reward is closely related to dopaminergic transmission which changes considerably due to synaptic pruning in the dopaminergic input of the prefrontal cortex (Rosenberg and Lewis, 1995). Therefore, the complex changes in the prefrontal-limbic system and the neurotransmitter systems associated with the maturation of this network, as noted earlier, make the adolescent brain unique and prone to misperceptions and miscalculations of risk (Kelley et al., 2004).

Caution is necessary when commenting on the developmental changes in brain activation during cognitive tasks. This is because task difficulty and performance significantly effects brain activation. Studies conducted with patients with schizophrenia showed that fMRI activation during working memory tasks indicated an inverted-U shaped function, meaning that both very easy and very difficult tasks resulted in lower activation (Callicott et al., 2003). In fact, poor performance may be due to failed performance in the engaged brain system or due to a brain system that is disengaged because of low performance or task design (Bullmore et al., 1999). This may also explain some of the discrepancies in former functional imaging studies, which are not consistent on whether cerebral activation increases or decreases with age for a given task. Three approaches are suggested to overcome the effect of difficulty: subject selection with different age groups showing similar behavioral performance; task selection with various levels of difficulty; and to computation of correlations netween age, cerebral activation, and age (Durston and Casey, 2006).

Adolescent brain may be more vulnerable to stress-related changes, because stress reactivity of the cerebral regions change with puberty. Moreover, adolescence is a high-risk period for stress exposure. Therefore, the combination of neurobiological vulnerability with increased environmental risk may lead to more prominent stress related changes in adolescent brain, particularly amygdala, hippocampus and prefrontal cortex. Romeo and McEwen (2004) stated that while the effect of stressors on adult hippocampus is reversible in adults, pubertal stress may not be so. Stress may have differential effects on adults and developing individuals. Prepubertal stress may effect sub-cortical structures while stress during adulthood have a greater impact on prefrontal cortex (Andersen et al., 2003). On the other hand, animal studies showed that favorable environmental conditions during adolescence may reverse the prior negative cerebral consequences of stress (Twiggs et al.,1978). Again, these results indicate that adolescence is both an important period of vulnerability and opportunity.

In summary, gray matter decrases with regional differences and white matter increases generally during adolescence. Synaptogenesis and synaptic pruning is seen during onset of puberty and adolescence, respectively. Synaptogenesis during puberty may lead to increased "interference" and lower cognitive performance, while the myelination and synaptic pruning lead to improvement in executive functions. Change of brain activation during development is complex and closely related to task difficulty and performance. Nevertheless, it can be concluded that with maturation brain activation becomes more focused and efficient. The increased capacity and efficiency during transition from adolescence to adulthood is related not only to maturation of individual brain regions, like prefrontal cortex, but to the maturation of the neural networks subserving improved abstract reasoning, decision making and executive control. Last of all, the high plasticity during adolescence may make the brain more susceptible to both development and vulnerability.

Neurobiology of Premorbid Schizophrenia: High-Risk and Prodromal Studies

As with other neuropsychiatric disorders, MRI studies have widely been used in schizophrenia research and have provided important results. Recent meta-analysis of volumetric MRI studies in schizophrenia suggest that global cerebral size is lower, ventricular volumes are higher and hippocampus-amygdala volumes are lower in subjects with schizophrenia (Wright et al., 2000; Shenton et al., 2000); however it is also suggested that the magnitude of structural difference of temporal cortex is too weak (Zakzanis et al., 2000; Davidson and Heinrichs, 2003). In another meta-analysis including only voxel-based morphometry studies left superior temporal gyrus and left medial temporal lobe emerged as key regions of structural difference in subjects with schizophrenia (Honea et al., 2005).

Studies conducted with first-episode psychotic subjects have the advantage to rule out possible drug and chronic disease effects. A recent meta-analysis of MRI studies conducted with first-episode schizophrenia subjects has indicated that the average sample sizes of these studies were smaller than those of subjects with chronic schizophrenia and that few findings were robustly significant (Steen et al., 2006). Whole-brain volumes of first-episode subjects were modestly (less than 3%) lower than the controls. Results of longitudinal studies suggested that the lateral ventricles were larger at firstdiagnosis. Hippocampus, planum temporale and temporal gray matter volumes were decreased at diagnosis and also showed continued volumetric loss during the course of the disorder, while volumetric changes in thalamus and insula seemed to be non-progressive. On the other hand, a large study of brain weight at autopsy showed that there were no correlations between brain weight and duration of psychosis (Harrison et al., 2003). Recently, a study using both auditory mismatch negativity (MMN, a bioelectric index of memory arising mainly from temporal cortex) and MRI reported that there might be an active period of "peri-onset cortical reduction" in schizophrenia (Salisbury et al., 2007). Results of this study indicated that in subjects with schizophrenia there was a close relationship between MMN amplitude and left Heschl gyrus gray matter volume, and both decreased during longitudinal follow-up, suggesting the presence of a late progressive lesion.

Some of the structural neroimaging studies also investigated the relation of cognitive variables with brain volumes. As summarized in a recent review (Antonova et al., 2004), these studies have found that total frontal lobe volume was correlated with executive function, working memory and verbal fluency performance in schizophrenia. Not all of these associations were evident in normal controls, presumably because of different degrees of variability in neuropsychological test performance depending on task difficulty and brain volumes. Some studies searched for association of neuropsychological test scores with specific regions of prefrontal cortex. These studies showed that gray matter volume of dorsolateral prefrontal cortex was related with better performance on tests measuring abstraction/flexibility and attention (Gur et al., 2000). Antonava et al (2004) further suggested that abnormalities in other brain regions might indeed contribute to impaired performance on neuropsychological tests purportedly related to prefrontal cortex functioning, like executive function, since prefrontal cortex is closely related with other brain regions (2004). In fact, it has been shown that hippocampal volumes were related with the performance in these tests. Results of two studies indicated that anterior hippocampal volumes were correlated with better executive functioning (Bilder et al., 1995; Szeszko et al., 2002). A very recent study showed that reduced volumes of the superior temporal gyrus and the fusiform gyrus volumes were related to positive symptoms-executive dysfunction and negative symptoms- facial memory deficits, respectively, suggesting a double-dissociation of anatomy and function in subjects with chronic schizophrenia (Nestor et al., 2007).

Since attention, working memory and executive functioning have been shown to be impaired in offspring of subjects with schizophrenia (Erlenmeyer-Kimling, 2000), the mentioned disturbances in prefrontal cortex in schizophrenia might include vulnerability factors present from childhood (Cannon et al., 2003). Impaired performance in working memory was found to be related with dorsolateral prefrontal structural abnormalities; furthermore, this relationship was associated with degree of genetic loading for schizophrenia (Cannon et al., 2002a, Glahn et al., 2002). Functional brain imaging studies have shown that both the subjects with schizophrenia and their relatives had reduced prefrontal perfusion (Blackwood et al., 1999). Finally, supporting evidence also comes from P300 and P50 studies: P300 and P50 abnormalities are among the most robust findings that discriminate between subjects with schizophrenia and normal controls (Bramon et al., 2004). These abnormalities have strong correlations with attentional and memory problems in subjects with schizophrenia and their first degree relatives (Yee et al. 1998; Shajahan et al., 1997; Blackwood et al., 1999), again pointing to the importance of attention problems in the emergence of this disorder.

In recent years, a growing number of studies have also investigated the structural brain alterations in relatives of schizohprenia probands. This is an important strategy allowing the researchers to study the trait and state factors related to schizophrenia. Although the results of these studies are not totally consistent, some suggestive patterns have emerged. Majority of these studies have shown that non-psychotic relatives of schizophrenia subjects have decreased hippocampus-amygdala (Lawrie et al., 1999; Keshavan et al., 2002; Seidman et al., 1999; O'Driscoll et al., 2001; Lawrie et al., 2001; vanErp et al., 2002; MacDonald et al., 2006), thalamus (Staal et al., 1998), and prefrontal cortex volumes (see Keshavan et al., 2002; Lawrie et al., 1999; Schreiber et al., 1999), increased lateral vetricles (Sharma et al., 1998; McDonald et al., 2002; but also Cannon et al., 1998; Lawrie et al., 1999; Seidman et al., 1999), and lack of normal cerebral asymmetry (Sharma et al., 1999; but Chapple et al., 2004). Some of the results suggested that the size of brain volumes of the relatives were between those of subjects and the normal controls, suggesting that the decrease in brain volumes may be related to genetic loading (Lawrie et al., 1999; McDonald et al., 2002; Staal et al., 1998; Sharma et al., 1999). A MRI study conducted with "ultra-high" risk individuals for schizophrenia found that those who developed psychosis (not schizophrenia) had decreased gray matter volumes in the right medial and lateral temporal cortex and inferior frontal cortex regions (Pantelis et al., 2003). Other studies found that gyrification abnormalities were evident in the right prefrontal lobe in the high-risk individuals who eventually developed shizophrenia (Harris et al., 2004); higher gray matter loss in right middle frontal gyrus was also reported (Job et al., 2003). The latter study also suggested that frontal-temporal cortices are important in the emergence of psychosis. A recent voxel-based morphometry study conducted with 35 individuals with an At Risk Mental State (ARMS) and first-episode subjects and controls showed that both ARMS and first-episode subjects had smaller gray matter volumes in left insula, superior temporal gyrus, in a midline region including posterior cingulate gyrus, and precuneus (Borgwardt et al., 2007). The ARMS patients that subsequently developed schizophrenia had smaller gray matter volume in the right insula, inferior frontal and superior temporal gyri. On the other hand parahippocampus, parietal and posterior temporal cortex and thalamus volumes were larger in the subjects that developed schizophrenia consistent with previous studies which suggested that transition to psychosis was related to progressive reduction in medial temporal volume (Job et al., 2005; Pantelis et al., 2003). Indeed, Job and associates reported that within the high-risk group significant declines in gray matter density were found in the temporal lobes, the right frontal lobe and right parietal lobe and those individuals at high risk who later developed schizophrenia also showed a different spatial pattern of reductions in the left temporal lobe and right cerebellum, from 2 to 3 years before they were diagnosed (2005). Not only structural but also functional differences may be evident in HR individuals. An fMRI study that compared ultra high-risk individuals, early and chronic schizophrenia subjects and controls during a visual oddball task paradigm reported that ultra-high-risk group showed smaller activation during task-relevant stimuli in the anterior cingulate, inferior frontal and medial frontal gyri than the control group. Both early and chronic groups had lower frontostriatal activation associated with target stimuli and the ultra-high-risk group showed a trend toward the early group. The authors concluded that prefrontal function might begin to decline before the onset of the disorder and prefrontal dysfunction might represent a vulnerability marker (Morey et al., 2005). However, not all studies found temporal cortex volume reductions in high-risk individuals (Schulze et al., 2003; Lawrie et al., 2002; Velakoulis et al., 2006). vanErp and associated showed that in the relatives hippocampal volume was related to genetic predisposition and fetal hypoxia, suggesting gene-environment iinteractions (van Erp et al., 2002). In a large sample, McDonald and associates suggested that hippocampal volume reduction is not endophenotypic for schizophrenia (2006). Thus, it is not clear whether hippocampus-amygdala volume reduction is a useful endophenotype of schizophrenia. In a recent review, DeLisi (2008) concluded that currently the studies are not consistent on which brain regions are abnormal during the prodromal period, onset, and first hospitalization.

Functional neuroimaging studies also explored the differences in relatives of schizophrenia patients. In adult relatives of schizophrenia subjects, exaggerated task-elicited activation in the prefrontal cortex has been reported (Callicott et al., 2003). In another study, researchers showed that first-degree relatives of schizophrenia had more cortical activity than controls in a wider set of prefrontal cortical regions during verbal encoding (Bonner-Jackson et al., 2007). In twin-pairs disconcordant for schizophrenia, Karlsgodt and associates (2007) reported that the un-affected co-twins' working memory (WM) performance and brain activation were intermediate between probands and controls, suggesting that the activation-performance relationship was disrupted both in the subjects and their unaffected relatives. Only a few studies have investigated the functional brain differences in younger HR individuals. An fMRI study with a very small sample size reported reduced activity during a spatial working memory task in the DLPFC (BA 8 and 9/46) and the inferior parietal cortex (BA 40) (Keshevan et al., 2002). In another study there was significantly higher activation in the left parietal lobe in HR subjects with psychotic symptoms that did not meet diagnostic criteria for psychotic disorder (Whalley et al., 2004). In a more recent study, in 21 non-psychotic relatives of individuals with schizophrenia Seidman and colleagues (2006) showed that young HR relatives had exaggerated brain activation in DLPFC during a working memory task suggesting that DLPFC processing during WM was inefficient in HR relatives. Authors also reported increased (although not statistically significant) activation in superior parietal lobule, which is connected with DLPFC and important in maintenance of attention (Corbetta et al., 2000). In a very recent study, 21 non-psychotic first-degree relatives with age range 13-28 were evaluated with fMRI during a verbal memory task (Thermenos et al., 2007). Results of that study indicated that the relatives had altered neural activity in parahipppocampus (in the entorhinal cortex region) during encoding despite normal performance. Two studies reported correlations between reduced hippocampal volume and verbal memory deficits in relatives (O'Driscoll et al., 2001; Seidman et al., 2002). However, the discussion above on the confounding factors of task difficulty and differences in task performance also applies to the summarized functional neuroimaging studies conducted with high-risk and schizophrenia samples. Nevertheless, it can be concluded that the patient and high-risk groups are inefficient in the use of cerebral resources and with increasing cognitive load they fail to increase cerebral activation as the healthy controls can do (Fusar-Poli et al., 2007).

Possible Links between Neurodevelopmental Changes in Adolescence and Onset of Schizophrenia

More than 25 years earlier, following his electrophysiology studies with psychotic adolescents, Feinberg (1982) suggested an association between synaptic elimination and the emergence of psychosis. Neuroimaging studies provided additonal support for the neurodevelopmental origin of schizophrenia, whereas numerous other studies suggested a progressive brain change theory in patients with schizophrenia (DeLisi, 2008). Temporal cortex, including hippocampus and amygdala, and prefrontal cortex are among the two brain regions that are implicated in the pathophysiology of schizophrenia. It has been also suggested that the changes in these two regions may be important in the emergence of psychosis. A number of MRI studies with high-risk groups showed that subjects with decreased temporal cortex and frontal cortex gray matter volumes might be at further risk of developing psychosis (Pantelis et al., 2003, Job et al., 2003, Borgwardt et al., 2007). These two regions mature relatively later and the increased connectivity between them may be necessary for the executive control of emotionally loaded conditions, which develops throughout the adolescence. Immaturity of this system may make adolescents more prone to stress related to reckless and impulsive behaviors and substance abuse, of which the developing adolescent brain is more susceptible to the unfavorable effects. In fact, the environmental adversities have additive effect on the persistence of psychotic symptoms in general population, suggesting that risk can also be reduced by decreasing the environmental load (Cougnard et al., 2007). Studies have shown that chronic exposure to glucocorticoids, hormones that are secreted in response to stress, is associated with hippocampal damage (reviewed in Thompson et al., 2004). Walker and Diforio (1997) suggested that in adolescence related increased activity in the HPA axis may lead to enhanced subcortical dopaminergic transmission in individuals who are pathologically sensitive to DA due to striatal receptor abnormalities. Hippocampus is also highly sensitive to the adverse effects of anoxia. Several studies have investigated whether pre-and perinatal risk factors were increased in subjects with schizophrenia. Meta-analytic studies reported that the obstetric complications are almost 2 times more common in patients with schizophrenia (Geddes and Lawrie, 1995). Obstetric complications may cause hypoxia-ischemia in the fetal brain. The ishemic damage due to fetal hypoxia may cause hippocampal damage that become more evident during the synaptic pruning of adolescence (Rosso et al., 2000).

In an oversimplification, we can think of an individual who is at increased risk of psychosis for various reasons (genetic loading, obstetric complications, and others) who has functional and structural brain differences, as well as reported cognitive, social, emotional and behavioral problems. The challenges brought by adolescence may lead to structural and functional changes in brain maturation in response to also to various environmental and social stresses as wel as related to risk-taking behaviors. The adolescent's resources (not only cognitive and behavioral but also neurodevelopmental) may not be adequate to face these challenges. Nonetheless, as discussed in previous sections, adolescence is also an important period of opportunity with growth of synaptogenesis during puberty that may makes the brain more sensitive to "experiential inputs" (Blakemore and Choudhury, 2006). Therefore, a multi-modal approach is necessary that includes a mix of measures: improved adult guidance, enriched social environments, and for individuals at particular high-risk, therapeutic interventions including use of medication, as may be useful, to help prevent emergence of psychosis.

Acknowledgment

This work supported by Fogarty/NIH D43 Grant TW05807 at Children's Hospital Boston (K.M.).

References

Adleman NE, Menon V, Blasey CM, White CD, Warsofsky IS, Glower GH, Reiss AL. (2002) A developmental fMRI study of the Stroop color-word task. *Neuroimage,* 16:61-75.

Andersen SL. (2003) Trajectories of brain development: point of vulnerability or window of opportunity? *Neuroscience and Biobehavioral Reviews,* 27:3-18.

Antonova E, Sharma T, Morris R, Kumari V. (2004) The relationship between brain structure and neurocognition in schizophrenia: a selective review. *Schizophr Res.* 70:117-45.

Benes FM, Turtle M, Khan Y, Farol P (1994). Myelination of a key relay zone in the hippocampal formation occurs in the human brain during childhood, adolescence, and adulthood. *Archives of General Psychiatry* 51:477-84.

Bilder RM, Bogerts B, Ashtari M, Wu H, Alvir JM, Jody D, Reiter G, Bell L,Lieberman JA. (1995) Anterior hippocampal volume reductions predict frontal lobe dysfunction in first episode schizophrenia. *Schizophr Res.*17:47-58.

Bjork JM, Knutson B, Fong GW, Caggiano DM, Bennett SM, Hommer DW (2004). Incentive-elicited brain activation in adolescents: similarities and differences from young adults. *Journal of Neuroscience,* 24:1793-1802.

Blackwood DH, Glabus MF, Dunan J, O'Carroll RE, Muir WJ, Ebmeier KP. (1999) Altered cerebral perfusion measured by SPECT in relatives of subjects with schizophrenia. Correlations with memory and P300.*Br J Psychiatry.* 175:357-66.

Blakemore S, Choudhury S. (2006) Development of the adolescent brain: implications for executive function and social cognition. *Journal of Child Psychology and Psychiatry,* 47:296-312.

Bonner-Jackson A, Csernansky JG, Barch DM. (2007) Levels-of-processing effects in first-degree relatives of individuals with schizophrenia. *Biol. Psychiatry.* 61:1141-7.

Borgwardt SJ, Riecher-Rossler A, Dazzan P, Chitnis X, Aston J, Drewe M, Gschwandtner U, Haller S, Pfluger M, Rechsteiner E, D'Souza M, Stieglitz RD, Radu EW, McGuire PK. (2007) Regional gray matter volume abnormalities in the at risk mental state. *Biol Psychiatry.* 61:1148-56.

Bourgeois JP, Goldman-Rakic PS, Rakic P. (1994) Synaptogenesis in the prefrontal cortex of rhesus monkey. *Cerebral Cortex,* 4:78-96.

Bramon E, Rabe-Hesketh S, Sham P, Murray RM, Frangou S. (2004) Meta-analysis of the P300 and P50 waveforms in schizophrenia.*Schizophr Res.* 70:315-29.

Bullmore E, Brammer M, Williams SC, Curtis V, McGuire P, Morris R, Murray R, Sharma T. (1999) Functional MR imaging of confounded hypofrontality. *Human Brain Mapping,* 8:86-91.

Bunge SA, Dudukovic NM, Thomason ME, Vaidya CJ, Gabrieli JD (2002) Immature frontal lobe contributions to cognitive control in children: evidence from fMRI. *Neuron,* 33:301-11.

Bunge SA, Wright SB. (2007) Neurodevelopmental changes in working memory and cognitive control. *Current Opinion in Neurobiology,* 17:243-50.

Callicott JH, Mattay VS, Verchinski BA, Marenco S, Egan MF,Weinberger DR. (2003) Complexity of prefrontal cortical dysfunction in schizophrenia: more than up or down. *Am J Psychiatry.* 160:2209-15.

Cannon TD, Thompson PM, van Erp TG, Toga AW, Poutanen VP, Huttunen M,Lonnqvist J, Standerskjold-Nordenstam CG, Narr KL, Khaledy M, Zoumalan I, Dail R, Kaprio J. (2002) Cortex mapping reveals regionally specific patterns of genetic and disease-specific gray-matter deficits in twins discordant for schizophrenia. *Proc Natl Acad Sci.* 99:3228-33.

Cannon TD, van Erp TG, Bearden CE, Loewy R, Thompson P, Toga AW, Huttunen MO, Keshavan MS, Seidman LJ, Tsuang MT. (2003) Early and late neurodevelopmental influences in the prodrome to schizophrenia:contributions of genes, environment, and their interactions. *Schizophr Bull.* 29:653-69

Cannon TD, van Erp TG, Huttunen M, Lonnqvist J, Salonen O, Valanne L,Poutanen VP, Standertskjold-Nordenstam CG, Gur RE, Yan M. (1998) Regional gray matter, white matter, and cerebrospinal fluid distributions in chizophrenic subjects, their siblings, and controls. *Arch Gen Psychiatry.* 55:1084-91.

Cannon TD, van Erp TG, Rosso IM, Huttunen M, Lonnqvist J, Pirkola T, Salonen O, Valanne L, Poutanen VP, Standertskjold-Nordenstam CG. (2002) Fetal hypoxia and structural brain abnormalities in schizophrenic subjects,their siblings, and controls.*Arch Gen Psychiatry.* 59:35-41.

Casey BJ, Trainor RJ, Orendi JL, Schubert AB, Nystrom LE, Cohen JD, Noll DC, Giedd J, Castellanos FX, Haxby J, Forman SD, Dahl RE, Rapoport JL (1997). A pediatric functional MRI study of prefrontal activation during performance of a Go-No-Go task. *Journal of Cognitive Neuroscience,* 9:835-47.

Caviness VS, Kennedy DN, Richelme C, Rademacher J, Filipek PA. (1996) The human brain age 7-11 years: a volmetric analysis based on magnetic resonance imaging. *Cerebral Cortex,* 6:726-36.

Chapple B, Grech A, Sham P, Toulopoulou T, Walshe M, Schulze K, Morgan K,Murray RM, McDonald C. (2004) Normal cerebral asymmetry in familial and non-familial schizophrenic probands sand their unaffected relatives. *Schizophr Res.*67:33-40.

Corbetta M, Kincade JM, Ollinger JM, McAvoy MP, Shulman GL.(2000) Voluntary orienting is dissociated from target detection in human posterior parietal cortex. *Nat Neurosci.* 3:292-7.

Cougnard A, Marcelis M, Myin-Germeys I, De Graaf R, Vollebergh W, Krabbendam L, Lieb R, Wittchen HU, Henquet C, Spauwen J, Van Os J. (2007) Does normal developmental expression of psychosis combine with environmental risk to cause persistence of psychosis? A psychosis proneness-persistence model. *Psychol Med.* 37:513-27.

Crews F, He J, Hodge C. (2007) Adolescent cortical development: a critical period of vulnerability for addiction. *Phamarcology, Biochemistry and Behavior,* 86:189-99.

Cunningham M, Bhattacharya GS, Benes FM (2002) Amygdalo-cortical sprouting continues into early adulthood: implications for the development of normal and abnormal function during adolescence. *Journal of Comparative Neurology* 453:116-130.

Dahl RE. (2004) Adolescent brain development: a period of vulnerabilities and opportunities. *Ann NY Acad Sci,* 1021:1-22.

Davidson LL, Heinrichs RW. (2003) Quantification of frontal and temporal lobe brain-imaging findings in schizophrenia: a meta-analysis. *Psychiatry Res.* 122:69-87.

DeLisi LE. (2008) The concept of progressive brain change in schizophrenia: implications for understanding schizophrenia. *Schizophr Bull.* 34:312-21.

Draganski B, Gaser C, Busch V, Schuierer G, Bogdahn U, May A.(2004) Neuroplasticity: changes in grey matter induced by training. *Nature.* 427:311-2.

Durston S, Casey BJ. (2006) What have we learned about cognitive development from neuroimaging? *Neuropsychologia.* 44:2149-57.

Durston S, Davidson MC, Tottenham N, Galvan A, Spicer J, Fosella JA, Casey BJ (2007). A shift from diffuse to focal cortical activity with development. *Dev Sci* 9:1-8.

Durston S, Davidson MC, Tottenham N, Galvan A, Spicer J, Fossella JA, Casey BJ. (2006) A shift from diffuse to focal cortical activity with development. *Dev Sci.*9:1-8.

Edin F, Macovenau J, Tegner J, Kingberg T. (2007) Stronger synaptic connectivity as a mechanism behind development of working memory related brain activity during childhood. *J Cog Neurosci,* 19; 750-60.

Feinberg I. (1982) Schizophrenia: caused by a fault in programmed synaptic elimination during adolescence? *J Psychiatr Res.*17:319-34.

Fusar-Poli P, Perez J, Broome M, Borgwardt S, Placentino A, Caverzasi E, Cortesi M, Veggiotti P, Politi P, Barale F, McGuire P. (2007) Neurofunctional correlates of vulnerability to psychosis: a systematic review and meta-analysis. *Neuroscience and Biobehavioral Reviews,* 31:465-84.

Gaillard WD, Hertz-Pannier L, Mott SH, Barnett AS, LeBihan D, Theodore WH (2000). Functional anatomy of cognitive development: fMRI of verbal fluency in children and adults. *Neurology,* 54:180-5.

Geddes JR, Lawrie SM. (1995) Obstetric complications and schizophrenia: a meta-analysis. Br J Psychiatry, 167;786-93.

Giedd JN, Blumenthal J, Jeffries NO, Castellanos FX, Liu H, Zijdenbos A, Paus T, Evans AC, Rapoport JL. (1999) Brain development during childhood and adolescence: a longitudinal MRI study. *Nature Neuroscience,* 2:861-3.

Giedd JN, Vaituzis AC, Vauss YC, Hamburger SD, Lange N, Rajapakse JC, Kaysen D, Vauss YC, Rapoport JL. (1996) Quantitative MRI of the temporal lobe, amygdala, and hippocampus in normal human development: ages 4-18 years. *Journal of Comparative Neurology* 366:223-30.

Glahn DC, Kim J, Cohen MS, Poutanen VP, Therman S, Bava S, Van Erp TG, Manninen M, Huttunen M, Lonnqvist J, Standertskjold-Nordenstam CG, Cannon TD. (2002) Maintenance and manipulation in spatial working memory: dissociations in the prefrontal cortex. *Neuroimage.* 17:201-13.

Gogtay N, Giedd JN, Lusk L, Hayashi KM, Greenstein D, Vaituzis AC, Nugent TF, Herman DH, Clasen LS, Toga AW, Rapoport JL, Thompson PM. (2004) Dynamic mapping of human cortical development during childhood through early adulthood. *Proceedings of the National Academy of Sciences of United States of America* 101:8174-9.

Gur RE, Cowell PE, Latshaw A, Turetsky BI, Grossman RI, Arnold SE, Bilker WB, Gur RC. (2000) Reduced dorsal and orbital prefrontal gray matter volumes in schizophrenia. *Arch Gen Psychiatry.* 57:761-8.

Harris JM, Whalley H, Yates S, Miller P, Johnstone EC, Lawrie SM. (2004) Abnormal cortical folding in high-risk individuals: a predictor of the development of schizophrenia? *Biol Psychiatry.* 56:182-9.

Harrison PJ, Freemantle N, Geddes JR. (2003) Meta-analysis of brain weight in schizophrenia. *Schizophr Res.* 64:25-34.

Honea R, Crow TJ, Passingham D, Mackay CE. (2005) Regional deficits in brain volume in schizophrenia: a meta-analysis of voxel-based morphometry studies. *Am J Psychiatry.* 162:2233-45.

Huttenlocher PR (1979) Synaptic density in human frontal cortex- developmental changes and effects of aging. *Brain Research,* 163:195-205.

Huttenlocher PR. (1984) Synapse elimination and plasticity in the developing human cerebral cortex. Am J Ment Defic 88:488-96.

Job DE, Whalley HC, Johnstone EC, Lawrie SM. (2005) Grey matter changes over time in high risk subjects developing schizophrenia.*Neuroimage.*25:1023-30.

Job DE, Whalley HC, McConnell S, Glabus M, Johnstone EC, Lawrie SM.

Karlsgodt KH, Glahn DC, van Erp TG, Therman S, Huttunen M, Manninen M, Kaprio J, Cohen MS, Lannqvist J, Cannon TD. (2007) The relationship between performance and fMRI signal during working memory in subjects with schizophrenia, unaffected co-twins, and control subjects. *Schizophr. Res* 89:191-7.

Kelley AE, Schochet T, Landry CF. (2004) Risk taking and novelty seeking in adolescence. *Ann NY Acad Sci,* 1021:27-32.

Keshavan MS, Dick E, Mankowski I, Harenski K, Montrose DM, Diwadkar V, DeBellis M. (2002) Decreased left amygdala and hippocampal volumes in young offspring at risk for schizophrenia. *Schizophr Res.* 58:173-83.

Killgore WDS, Yurgelun-Todd DA (2007) Neural correlates of emotional intelligence in adolescent children. *Cognitive, Affective and Behavioral Neuroscience,* 7:140-51.

Lawrie SM, Whalley H, Kestelman JN, Abukmeil SS, Byrne M, Hodges A,Rimmington JE, Best JJ, Owens DG, Johnstone EC. (1999) Magnetic resonance imaging of brain in people at high risk of developing schizophrenia. *Lancet.* 1999;35330-3.

Lawrie SM, Whalley HC, Abukmeil SS, Kestelman JN, Donnelly L, Miller P,Best JJ, Owens DG, Johnstone EC. (2001) Brain structure, genetic liability, and psychotic symptoms in subjects at high risk of developing schizophrenia.*Biol Psychiatry.* 49:811-23.

Lawrie SM, Whalley HC, Abukmeil SS, Kestelman JN, Miller P, Best JJ, Owens DG, Johnstone EC. (2002) Temporal lobe volume changes in people at high risk of schizophrenia with psychotic symptoms. *Br J Psychiatry.* 181:138-43.

Lenroot RK, Giedd JN. (2006) Brain development in children and adolescents: insight from anatomical magnetic resonance imaging. *Neuroscience and Biobehavioral Reviews,* 30:718-29.

Lenroot RK, Schmitt JE, Ordaz SJ, Wallace GL, Neale MC, Lerch JP, Kendler KS, Evans AC, Giedd JN. (2007) Differences in genetic and environmental influences on the human cerebral cortex associated with development during childhood and adolescence. *Hum Brain Mapp.*

Luna B, Sweeney JA (2004) The emergence of collaborative brain function: fMRI studies of the development of response inhibition. *Ann NY Acad Sci,* 1021:296-309.

MacDonald AW, Becker TM, Carter CS. (2006) Functional magnetic resonance imaging study of cognitive control in the healthy relatives of schizophrenia subjects. *Biol. Psychiatry.* 60:1241-9.

McDonald C, Marshall N, Sham PC, Bullmore ET, Schulze K, Chapple B, Bramon E, Filbey F, Quraishi S, Walshe M, Murray RM.(2006) Regional brain morphometry in subjects with schizophrenia or bipolar disorder and their unaffected relatives. *Am J Psychiatry.* 163:478-87.

McGivern RF, Andersen J, Byrd D, Mutter KL, Reilly J. (2002) Cognitive efficiency on a match to sample task decreases at the onset of puberty in children. *Brain and Cognition,* 50:73-89.

Mesulam MM. (2000) A plasticity-based theory of the pathogenesis of Alzheimer's disease. *Ann NY Acad Sci,* 924:42-52.

Morey RA, Inan S, Mitchell TV, Perkins DO, Lieberman JA, Belger A. (2005) Imaging frontostriatal function in ultra-high-risk, early, and chronic schizophrenia during executive processing.*Arch Gen Psychiatry*. 62:254-62.

Nestor PG, Kubicki M, Spencer KM, Niznikiewicz M, McCarley RW, Shenton ME. (2007) Attentional networks and cingulum bundle in chronic schizophrenia. *Schizophr Res.* 90:308-15.

Nestor PG, Onitsuka T, Gurrera RJ, Niznikiewicz M, Frumin M, Shenton ME, McCarley RW. (2007) Dissociable contributions of MRI volume reductions of superior temporal and fusiform gyri to symptoms and neuropsychology in schizophrenia. *Schizophr Res.* 91:103-6.

O'Driscoll GA, Florencio PS, Gagnon D, Wolff AV, Benkelfat C, Mikula L, Lal S, Evans AC. (2001) Amygdala-hippocampal volume and verbal memory in first-degree relatives of schizophrenic subjects. *Psychiatry Res.* 107:75-85.

Pantelis C, Velakoulis D, McGorry PD, Wood SJ, Suckling J, Phillips LJ, Yung AR, Bullmore ET, Brewer W, Soulsby B, Desmond P, McGuire PK. (2003) Neuroanatomical abnormalities before and after onset of psychosis: a cross-sectional and longitudinal MRI comparison. *Lancet.* 361:281-8.

Romeo RD, McEwen BS. (2004) *Stress and the adolescent brain.* Ann NY Acad Sci, 1021:202-14.

Rosenberg DR, Lewis DA. (1995) Postnatal maturation of the dopaminergic innervation of monkey prefrontal and motor cortices: a tyrosine hydroxylase immunohistochemical analysis. *J Comp Neurology,* 358:383-400.

Rosso IM, Cannon TD, Huttunen T, Huttunen MO, LOnnqvist J, Gasperoni TL. (2000) Obstetric risk factors for early-onset schizophrenia in a Finnish birth cohort. *Am J Psychiatry,* 157;801-807.

Salisbury DF, Kuroki N, Kasai K, Shenton ME, McCarley RW. (2007) Progressive and interrelated functional and structural evidence of post-onset brain reduction in schizophrenia. *Arch Gen Psychiatry.*64:521-9.

Schlaggar BL, Brown TT, Lugar HM, Visscher KM, Mlezin FM, Petersen SE. (2002) Functional neuroanatomical differences between adults and school-age children in the processing of single words. *Science,* 296:1476-1479.

Schreiber H, Baur-Seack K, Kornhuber HH, Wallner B, Friedrich JM, De Winter IM, Born J. (1999) Brain morphology in adolescents at genetic risk for schizophrenia assessed by qualitative and quantitative magnetic resonance imaging. *Schizophr Res.* 40:81-4.

Schulze K, McDonald C, Frangou S, Sham P, Grech A, Toulopoulou T,Walshe M,Sharma T, Sigmundsson T, Taylor M, Murray RM. (2003) Hippocampal volume in familial and nonfamilial schizophrenic probands and their unaffected relatives.*Biol Psychiatry.* 53:562-70.

Seidman LJ, Faraone SV, Goldstein JM, Goodman JM, Kremen WS, Toomey R,Tourville J, Kennedy D, Makris N, Caviness VS, Tsuang MT. (1999) Thalamic and amygdala-hippocampal volume reductions in first-degree relatives of patients with schizophrenia: an MRI-based morphometric analysis.*Biol Psychiatry.* 46:941-54.

Seidman LJ, Thermenos HW, Poldrack RA, Peace NK, Koch JK, Faraone SV, Tsuang MT. (2006) Altered brain activation in dorsolateral prefrontal cortex in adolescents and young adults at genetic risk for schizophrenia: an fMRI study of working memory. *Schizophr Res.*85:58-72.

Shajahan PM, O'Carroll RE, Glabus MF, Ebmeier KP, Blackwood DH. (1997) Correlation of auditory 'oddball' P300 with verbal memory deficits in schizophrenia. *Psychol Med.* 27:579-86.

Sharma T, Lancaster E, Lee D, Lewis S, Sigmundsson T, Takei N, Gurling H, Barta P, Pearlson G, Murray R. (1998) Brain changes in schizophrenia. Volumetric MRI study of families multiply affected with schizophrenia--the Maudsley Family Study 5. *Br J Psychiatry.* 173:132-8.

Sharma T, Lancaster E, Sigmundsson T, Lewis S, Takei N, Gurling H, Barta P,Pearlson G, Murray R. (1999) Lack of normal pattern of cerebral asymmetry in familial schizophrenic subjects and their relatives – The Maudsley Family Study. *Schizophr Res.* 40:111-20.

Shaw P, Greenstein D, Lerch J, Clasen L, Lenroot R, Gogtay N (2006) Intellectual ability and cortical development in children and adolescents. *Nature,* 440:676-9.

Shenton ME, Dickey CC, Frumin M, McCarley RW. (2001) A review of MRI findings in schizophrenia. *Schizophr Res.* 49:1-52.

Sisk CL, Foster DL. (2004) The neural basis of puberty and adolesence. *Nature Neuroscience,* 7:1040-7.

Sowell ER, Thompson PM, Leonard CM, Welcome SE, Kan E, Toga AW (2004) Longitudinal mapping of cortical thickness and brain growth in normal children. *Journal of Neuroscience,* 24:8223-31.

Sowell ER, Peterson BS, Thompson PM, Welcome SE, Henkenius AL, Toga AW. (2003) Mapping cortical change across the life-span. *Nature Neuroscience.* 6:309-15.

Sowell ER, Thompson PM, Holmes CJ, Batth R, Jernigan TL, Toga AW. (1999) Localizing age related changes in brain structure between childhood and adolescence using statistical parametric mapping. *Neuroimage,* 6:587-97.

Sowell ER, Thompson PM, Tessner KD, Toga AW. (2001) Mapping continued brain growth and gray matter density reduction in dorsal frontal cortex: inverse relationships during postadolescent brain maturation. *Journal of Neuroscience,* 21:8819-29.

Spessot AL, Plessen KJ, Peterson BS. (2004) Neuroimaging of developmental psychopathologies: the importance of self-regulatory and neuroplastic processes in adolescence. *Ann NY Acad Sci,* 1021:86-104.

Staal WG, Hulshoff Pol HE, Schnack H, van der Schot AC, Kahn RS. (1998) Partial volume decrease of the thalamus in relatives of subjects with schizophrenia. *Am J Psychiatry.* 155:1784-6.

Steen RG, Mull C, McClure R, Hamer RM, Lieberman JA. (2006) Brain volume in first-episode schizophrenia: systematic review and meta-analysis of magnetic resonance imaging studies. *Br J Psychiatry.*188:510-8.

Szeszko PR, Strous RD, Goldman RS, Ashtari M, Knuth KH, Lieberman JA, Bilder RM. (2002) Neuropsychological correlates of hippocampal volumes in subjects experiencing a first episode of schizophrenia. *Am J Psychiatry.* 159:217-26.

Thermenos HW, Seidman LJ, Poldrack RA, Peace NK, Koch JK, Faraone SV, Tsuang MT. (2007) Elaborative verbal encoding and altered anterior parahippocampal activation in adolescents and young adults at genetic risk for schizophrenia using FMRI. *Biol. Psychiatry.*61:564-74.

Thompson JL, Pogue-Geile MF, Grace AA. (2004) Developmental pathology, dopamine, and stress: a model for the age of onset of schizophrenia symptoms. *Schizophr Bull.* 30:875-900.

Toga AW, Thompson PM, Sowell ER. (2006) Mapping brain maturation. *Trends in Neuroscience,* 29:148-59.

Twigs DG, Popolow HB, Gerall AA.(1978) Medial preoptic lesions and male sexual behavior: age and environmental interactions. *Science,* 200:1414-5.

Van Erp TG, Saleh PA, Rosso IM, Huttunen M, Lönnqvist J, Pirkola T, Salonen O,Valanne L, Poutanen VP, Standertskjöld-Nordenstam CG, Cannon TD. (2002) Contributions of genetic risk and fetal hypoxia to hippocampal volume in patients with schizophrenia or schizoaffective disorder, their unaffected siblings, and healthy unrelated volunteers. *Am J Psychiatry.* 159:1514-20.

Velakoulis D, Wood SJ, Wong MT, McGorry PD, Yung A, Phillips L, Smith D,Brewer W, Proffitt T, Desmond P, Pantelis C. (2006) Hippocampal and amygdala volumes according to psychosis stage and diagnosis: a magnetic resonance imaging study of chronic schizophrenia, first-episode psychosis, and ultra-high-risk individuals. *Arch Gen Psychiatry.*63:139-49.

Volpe JJ. (2000) Overview: normal and abnormal human brain development. *Mental Retardation and Developmental Disabilities Research Reviews* 6:1-5.

Voxel-based morphometry of grey matter densities in subjects at high risk of schizophrenia. *Schizophr Res.* 2003;64:1-13.

Walker EF, Diforio D (1997) Schizophrenia: a neural diathesis-stress model.*Psychol Rev.*104:667-85.

Weiss EM, Siedentopf C, Golaszewski S, Mottaghy FM, Hofer A, Kremser C, Felber S, Fleischhacker WW. (2007) Brain activation patterns during a selective attention test--a functional MRI study in healthy volunteers and unmedicated subjects during an acute episode of schizophrenia. *Psychiatry Res.* 154:31-40.

Whalley HC, Simonotto E, Flett S, Marshall I, Ebmeier KP, Owens DG, Goddard NH, Johnstone EC, Lawrie SM. (2004) fMRI correlates of state and trait effects in subjects at genetically enhanced risk of schizophrenia. *Brain.* 127:478-90.

Wright IC, Rabe-Hesketh S, Woodruff PW, David AS, Murray RM, Bullmore ET. (2000) Meta-analysis of regional brain volumes in schizophrenia. *Am J Psychiatry.* 157:16-25.

Yakovlev PA, Lecours IR (1967) The myelogenetic cycles of regional maturation of the brain. In A. Minkowski (Ed), *Regional development of the brain in early life* (pp.3-70). Oxford, Blackwell.

Yee CM, Nuechterlein KH, Morris SE, White PM. (1998) P50 suppression in recent-onset schizophrenia: clinical correlates and risperidone effects. *J Abnorm Psychol.* 107:691-8.

Zakzanis KK, Poulin P, Hansen KT, Jolic D. (2000) Searching the schizophrenic brain for temporal lobe deficits: a systematic review and meta-analysis. *Psychol Med* 30:491-504.

In: Adolescent Schizophrenia
Editors: J. T. Nillinghouse and R. P. Trotman
ISBN: 978-1-60692-370-2

Chapter II

The Association of Visuospatial Memory and Working Memory with Adolescent Onset Schizophrenia

Alasdair Vance [*]
Head Academic Child Psychiatry, Department of Paediatrics, University of Melbourne
Murdoch Childrens Research Institute, Royal Children's Hospital, Parkville, Melbourne
VIC 3052, Australia

Abstract

This chapter investigates the nature of and association between visuospatial memory, and, separately, visuospatial working memory in adolescent onset schizophrenia. The data presented suggest that both the visuospatial memory and working memory performance of the adolescent-onset schizophrenia group are impaired compared to the healthy control group. Further, the type and magnitude of the deficits are similar to those reported in the adult-onset schizophrenia patients suggesting these deficits are developmental stage independent. The import of these findings is examined within the context of emerging neurobiological models of progressive parietal-temporal-frontal linked neural network dysfunction in schizophrenia, whether of adolescent- or adult-onset. Also, the implications of these findings for the current aetiological understanding of schizophrenia and the current assessment and treatment approaches are discussed.

[*] Phone: 61 3 9345-4666; Fax: 61 3 9345-6002; email: avance@unimelb.edu.au

Introduction

It is known that the cognitive neuroscience constructs of visuospatial memory and working memory are associated with adult- and adolescent-onset schizophrenia. However, to date, the specific associations between well defined measures of visuospatial memory and visuospatial working memory, with known brain behaviour relationships, and carefully defined adolescent onset schizophrenia have not been studied. This chapter reviews the extant literature and explores the nature of and association between visuospatial memory, and, separately, visuospatial working memory in adolescent onset schizophrenia. Data from the cross sectional comparison of adolescent onset schizophrenia with a healthy control group, matched for age, gender and fullscale IQ on the above cognitive neuroscience measures are presented. Both the visuospatial memory and working memory performance of the adolescent-onset schizophrenia group are impaired compared to the healthy control group. Further, the type and magnitude of the deficits are similar to those reported in the adult-onset schizophrenia patients suggesting these deficits are developmental stage independent. The import of these findings is examined within the context of emerging neurobiological models of progressive parietal-temporal-frontal linked neural network dysfunction in schizophrenia, whether of adolescent- or adult-onset. Also, the implications of these findings for the current aetiological understanding of schizophrenia and the current assessment and treatment approaches are discussed.

Study 1

Visuospatial memory deficits are replicated findings in adults (Bilder et al., 2000) and adolescents (Kravariti et al., 2003; Rhinewine et al., 2005) with schizophrenia and those at risk for developing schizophrenia (Brewer et al., 2005; Smith et al., 2006). The magnitude of these deficits ranges between 1-2 standard deviations (Rhinewine et al., 2005) and they are qualitatively similar (Kravariti et al., 2003; Rund et al., 2004). To date, in adults and adolescents with schizophrenia, visuospatial memory deficits have been investigated primarily through the parsing of visuospatial working memory into its maintenance and manipulation components: both of these subprocesses have been found to be deficient in adults (Cannon et al., 2005) and adolescents (Wood et al., 2003; Mathes et al., 2005) with schizophrenia. Also, manipulation abilities are more severely affected than maintenance aspects in visuospatial (Cannon et al., 2005) and verbal (Tan et al., 2005) working memory. Further, the encoding aspect of visuospatial memory, within the broader visuospatial working memory construct, has been specifically implicated (Fleming et al., 1997; Hartman et al., 2002; Liederman and Strejilovich, 2004), while encoding or storage processes have been associated with increasing genetic predisposition to schizophrenia (Glahn et al., 2003).

The delayed matching-to-sample (DMTS) task from the Cambridge Neuropsychological Test Automated Battery (CANTAB) (Owen et al., 1996) is able to readily parse out encoding from retrieval aspects of visuospatial memory for the following reasons: Firstly, the memory demand of the test can be increased by extending the delay between the offset of the target stimulus and the onset of the exemplars. Increasing the delay makes the representation of the encoded stimulus vulnerable to decay, placing greater demand on retrieval processes (Paule et al., 1998). Secondly, by presenting the choice exemplars while the target stimuli remains visible (a matching to sample task (MTS)) the memory demand of the task can be eliminated. The MTS condition provides an ideal control to determine the extent to which factors influencing encoding, such as perceptual discrimination differences, may contribute to later deficits in the recognition or recall of target stimuli (Pantelis et al., 2001). Manipulation of the exemplars such that they share some, but not all, of the target features (for example, the same shape as the target but a different colour) allows the analysis of the types of strategies used by subjects to make decisions based on memory (Owen et al., 1995). Because responses to the DMTS task can be made manually and pictorial stimuli can be used, the extent to which any language impairment alters performance is reduced. Finally, the simultaneous and delayed task conditions are randomized, with all conditions identical until after stimulus presentation (Barnett et al., 2005; Mathes et al., 2005).

However, to date, investigation of DMTS performance in adults with early phase and chronic adult-onset schizophrenia has revealed encoding deficits (Mathes et al., 2005), while encoding and retrieval deficits have been suggested in first episode adult-onset schizophrenia and those at risk for adult-onset schizophrenia (Wood et al., 2003). Given the patients with schizophrenia in the latter study were younger and Luciana et al. (2005) have reported that healthy adolescents aged 16 years and over have significantly better DMTS performance than 13-15 year old healthy adolescents, the encoding and retrieval deficits in the younger patients with schizophrenia may be developmental stage dependent: specifically, the encoding deficits may be contributing to the retrieval deficits in the younger patients rather than there being independent retrieval deficits. This study investigates whether the encoding and/or retrieval phases of visuospatial memory are impaired in carefully defined adolescents with schizophrenia. We hypothesize that that there will be encoding deficits alone, consistent with findings in adults with schizophrenia.

Method

Participants

Nineteen right-handed male adolescents aged 12-17 years [14.64 (1.85) years] were identified with medication naïve, undifferentiated schizophrenia (DSM-IV, American Psychiatric Association, 1994) during their initial clinical evaluation before active treatment (Vance et al., 2007). This was defined through a semi-structured clinical interview *(Schedule for Affective Disorders and Schizophrenia – childhood version (K-SADS)*, Kaufman et al., 1997) with their parent(s) and with each adolescent ($\kappa > 0.80$) and by the clinician-completed *Positive and Negative Symptom Scale (PANSS)* (Kay et al., 1987): *Positive Scale* score of mean 67.11 (23.29) (percentile), a *Negative Scale* score of 79.53 (20.71) (percentile) and a *General Psychopathological Scale* score of 89.95 (21.30) (percentile). The undifferentiated schizophrenia group had a fullscale IQ of 109.10 (15.00) (*Wechsler Intelligence Scale for Children (WISC-3)* (Wechsler, 1991), with all fullscale IQs above 80 and a duration of illness of mean 12.45 (3.67) months. All the group were living in a family home and attending normal schools and none had overt neurological or endocrine disease or colour blindness. Twenty eight healthy male control participants were recruited through local schools, who did not meet criteria for any psychiatric, neurological or endocrine disorder, again defined through a semi-structured clinical interview *(K-SADS)*, Kaufman et al., 1997) with their parent(s) and with each adolescent and by the clinician-completed *PANSS* [(Kay et al., 1987): *Positive Scale* score of 2.11 (0.57) (percentile); $t(45) = 14.83$, $p < 0.0005$, a *Negative Scale* score of 1.71 (0.81) (percentile); $t(45) = 19.97$, $p < 0.0005$ and a *General Psychopathological Scale* score of 1.04 (0.19) (percentile); $t(45) = 22.20$, $p < 0.0005$] and who did not differ from the undifferentiated schizophrenia group in age [13.47 (1.77); $t(45) = 1.58$, $p = 0.12$) and fullscale IQ [105.89 (6.92); $t(45) = 0.98$, $p = 0.33$].

Measures

Visuospatial memory was assessed through measurement of performance on the DMTS task selected from the CANTAB (Owen et al., 1996). The computerised test was presented on a high resolution IBM monitor with a touch sensitive screen. All participants reported previous experience with computers. The DMTS test assessed the ability to recall a complex target stimulus (an abstract pattern), presented on the screen for 4 seconds. There were four conditions, each with 10 trials presented randomly. In the MTS condition, the target stimulus remained on the screen with the choice exemplars. In the delay conditions, the target stimulus was removed followed by a 0, 4 or 12 second delay before the choice exemplars were presented. In all trials, subjects were required to choose the target stimulus in a four-alternative forced choice procedure between the correct pattern, and three 'distractor' patterns. Performance was measured according to the percentage of correct responses at the simultaneous and each of the delay levels. Further analysis examined three types of possible errors at each level of the task. 1) a "colour error" was committed when the subject selected the wrong coloured pattern but the correct shape; 2) a "shape error" was committed when the subject selected an incorrectly shaped pattern that was the correct colour, and 3) an "unrelated error" was committed when the incorrect pattern was selected that was both the wrong colour and shape (Barnett et al., 2005).

Statistical Analysis

Latencies for the DMTS task were transformed using logarithmic (base 10) transformations to reduce skewness in the distribution (Maruff et al., 1996). Performance on the DMTS task was compared with a repeated measures multivariate analysis of covariance (MANCOVA) using a two-factor design that included a between-subjects factor (group) and a within subjects factor (delay level), co-varying for the effects of age and fullscale IQ, given the known sensitivity of visuospatial memory measures to these variables (Kravariti et al., 2003; Barnett et al., 2005). To protect against violation of the homogeneity of covariance assumption, analysis of within-group effects or interactions with degrees of freedom greater than one were examined using a repeated measures design within MANCOVA (Wilk's

Multivariate test of significance) (Tabachnick and Fidell, 2001). MANCOVA was also performed to analyse the accuracy and latency across delay conditions, covarying for performance on the MTS condition in addition to age and fullscale IQ. To estimate effect sizes, Cohen's *d* calculation for unequal sample sizes was used (Zakzanis, 2001) to examine differences between group performance on both accuracy and latency measures. In order to protect against a type 1 error, the level of significance for comparisons was set at 0.01. For the number of each type of error made on the DMTS task, the number of each error type made by each subject at each level of the test was submitted to a 2 (group) x 4 (condition) x 3 (error type) repeated measures MANCOVA, with error type as an additional within subject variable, again co-varying for the effects of age and fullscale IQ. Finally, the relationship between response accuracy and response latency, covarying for the effects of age and fullscale IQ, was explored using Pearson product moment correlation coefficients. This same procedure was also used to assess the strength of the relationship between participants' DMTS task performance accuracy, severity of psychotic symptoms (PANSS) and levels of inattention (Child Behaviour Checklist, attention subscale) (Achenbach, 1991), given the known strong association between inattention and memory encoding difficulties (Devilbiss et al., 2006).

Results

Figure 1 shows the group mean percentage correct accuracy of performance and Table 1 the comparison of accuracy rates between the two groups on all conditions of the DMTS test. MANCOVA indicated a significant effect of group [$F(1,43)=18.92$, $p<0.0005$] after controlling for age and full-scale IQ, only the former having a significant independent association with the DMTS accuracy variables [$F(1,43)=28.33$, $p<0.0005$]. When averaged across all four conditions, the control group [88.40 (2.93)] made fewer errors than the undifferentiated schizophrenia group [(80.53 (4.14)]. Figure 2 (filled bar) shows the effect size for this comparison. The MANCOVA also indicated a significant effect of condition [Wilk's $\lambda=0.68$, $F(3,41)=6.36$, $p=0.001$]. There was also a significant group x condition interaction [Wilk's $\lambda=0.75$, $F(3, 41)=4.56$, $p=0.008$], after controlling for age [Wilk's $\lambda=0.69$, $F(3, 41)=6.25$, $p=0.001$], and full-scale IQ [Wilk's $\lambda=0.77$, $F(3, 41)=3.99$, $p=0.01$], both of which had a significant independent association with the DMTS accuracy variables.

To determine the extent to which differences between groups in the accuracy of encoding information affected the accuracy of their recall after a delay, the group x condition MANCOVA was repeated with the three DMTS conditions entered as levels of the independent variable and accuracy on the MTS condition treated as a covariate. This analysis indicated that the covariate was non-significant [$F(1, 42)=1.17$, $p=0.29$], with the effect of group remaining significant when the effect of the covariate was removed [$F(1, 42)=14.10$, $p=0.001$], as did the effect of condition [Wilks $\lambda=0.73$, $F(2, 41)=7.62$, $p=0.002$]. Effect size (Cohen's *d*) for the corrected difference between conditions is shown in Figure 2 (unfilled bar). This Figure illustrates that the magnitude of the group differences across delay conditions was reduced by approximately 23% with the accuracy of performance on MTS trials removed. The interaction between group and condition became non-significant with the covariate added to the analysis [Wilks λ=0.84, $F(2, 41)=3.96, p=0.03$].

For response latency, MANCOVA indicated a non-significant effect of group [$F(1,43)=1.06$, $p=0.31$] [control group 3.55 (0.10) s; undifferentiated schizophrenia group 3.52 (0.12) s] and condition [Wilk's λ=.84 $F(3, 41)=2.63$, $p=0.06$]. After controlling for age and fullscale IQ, both of which had no significant independent association with DMTS latency variables, there was a significant group x condition interaction [Wilk's λ=0.66, $F(3, 41)=6.95$, $p=0.001$].

To determine the extent to which differences between groups in the speed of encoding information affected the speed of their recall after a delay, the group x condition MANCOVA was repeated with the log 10 latencies for each subject as the dependent variable and the three DMTS conditions entered as levels of the repeated factor and log 10 latencies on the MTS condition treated as a covariate. This analysis indicated that the covariate was significant [$F(1, 42)=23.15$, $p<0.0005$]. The effect of group became significant with the effect of the covariate removed [$F(1, 42)=7.34$, $p<0.01$]. The effect of condition remained non-significant with the covariate removed [Wilks λ=0.95, $F(2, 41)=1.15$, $p=0.33$], although, as Figure 2 shows, the effect size for the difference between groups altered substantially with the covariate removed (unfilled bar). The interaction between group and condition remained significant with the covariate added to the analysis [Wilks Lambda=0.70, $F(2, 41)=8.85$, $p=0.001$], after controlling for age and full-scale IQ, both of which had no significant independent association with DMTS latency variables.

For analysis of error type, MANCOVA indicated a significant main effect of group [$F(1,42)=18.09$, $p<0.0005$]. As the differences between groups for the mean number of errors, averaged across all error types, is the inverse of the finding of differences between groups for accuracy of performance (shown above), this effect was not explored further. MANCOVA also indicated a significant main effect for condition [Wilk's λ=0.63, $F(3,40)=7.56$, $p<0.0005$], while error type and condition x error type interaction were non-significant.

For the MTS condition, no significant correlations were found between response accuracy and Log10 latency of correct responses in the control [$r=0.22$, $p=0.27$] or undifferentiated schizophrenia [$r=-0.03$, $p=0.90$] groups. No significant correlation was found between accuracy on the delay conditions (percentage correct averaged across 0, 4 and 12 second delay conditions) and latency for the control [$r=0.15$, $p=0.46$] or undifferentiated schizophrenia [$r=0.40$, $p=0.09$] groups.

No significant correlations were found between DMTS task performance and positive [$r=-0.30$, $p=0.16$] or negative [$r=-0.45$, $p=0.11$] psychotic symptom severity or levels of inattention [$r=-0.28$, $p=0.27$] in the undifferentiated schizophrenia group. Similarly, no significant correlations were found between DMTS task performance and positive [$r=-0.24$, $p=0.25$] or negative[$r=-0.16$, $p=0.42$] psychotic symptom severity or levels of inattention [$r=-0.22$, $p=0.27$] in the control group.

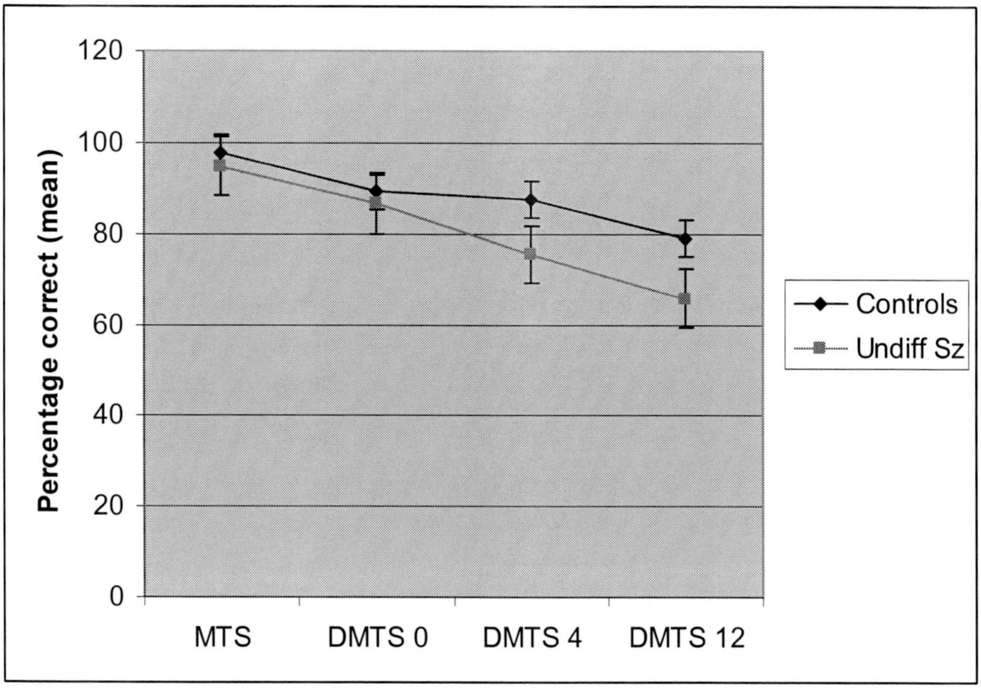

Figure 1. Response accuracy of each group at each condition of the DMTS task.

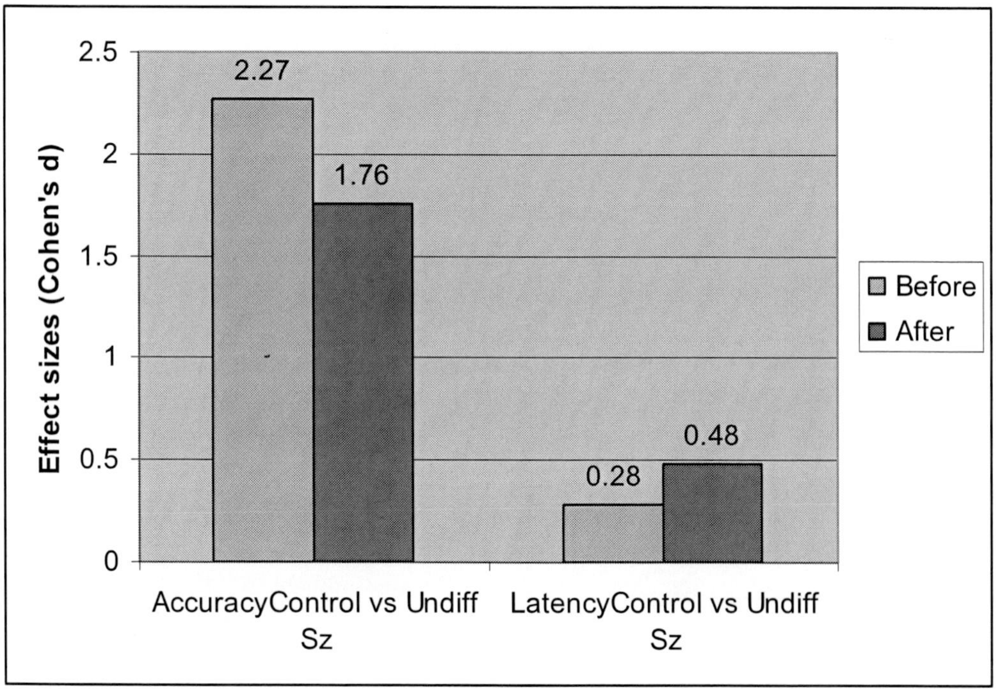

Figure 2. Effect sizes before and after covarying for performance on the MTS condition.

Table 1. Comparison of accuracy rates across each condition of the delayed-matching-to sample test

	Controls N = *28* **Mean (SD)**	**Sz** N = *19* **Mean (SD)**	*p*
MTS trials (% correct)	97.86 (6.30)	94.74 (8.41)	0.15
DMTS 0 second delay (% correct)	89.29 (13.03)	86.32 (13.00)	0.45
DMTS 4 second delay (% correct)	87.50 (12.95)	75.26 (20.65)	0.02
DMTS12 second delay (% correct)	78.93 (14.49)	65.79 (24.11)	0.02
DMTS delay trials (% correct averaged across delay trials only)	85.24 (11.84)	75.79 (17.24)	0.03

Controls: healthy control participants. Sz: undifferentiated schizophrenia participants.

Discussion

Anti-psychotic medication naïve adolescents with undifferentiated schizophrenia demonstrated subtle yet significant impairment in performance on a visuospatial memory test. Although performance on the memory test was generally worse in the undifferentiated schizophrenia group than the healthy control participants, the pattern of decrease in overall accuracy from the MTS to the 12 second DMTS condition was qualitatively similar in both groups (Figure 1). Further, although accuracy decreased substantially from the MTS to DMTS conditions for both groups, they could not be differentiated statistically across the 0 to 4 second and from the 4 to 12 second delay conditions. When the 'visible exemplar' condition (MTS) and the 'removed from view' exemplar conditions (DMTS) were examined together, an interaction effect was obtained suggesting that the undifferentiated schizophrenia group behaved differently to the healthy control participants across these stages. However, this interaction effect disappeared when DMTS performance between the two groups was examined covarying for the MTS performance. Taken together, these findings suggest that the undifferentiated schizophrenia group are generally worse at remembering the exemplars but not at any particular delay. Also, although the medication naïve adolescents with undifferentiated schizophrenia were significantly faster at responding on the delay conditions than the healthy control participants, there was no correlation between the speed of response and accuracy of DMTS task performance in either group. Further, error type did not differ between the two groups on the MTS and delay conditions. Hence, the difference between DMTS task performance between the two groups is unlikely to be due to motivational differences and/or manifestly different approaches to task completion. In particular, the adolescents with undifferentiated schizophrenia appear to be using the same decision making strategy, obeying the task rules, adhering to the task requirements and not selecting targets at random (Barnett et al., 2005). Similarly, the absence of any correlation between the level of psychotic symptoms, level of inattention and DMTS task performance in either group suggests that the DMTS performance impairments in the undifferentiated schizophrenia group are not secondary to these behavioural symptoms.

These findings are consistent with the adolescents with undifferentiated schizophrenia experiencing an encoding impairment rather than a problem with retrieval (Barnett et al., 2005). Consequently, poorer performance during the delay conditions of the task may have occurred because the adolescents with undifferentiated schizophrenia had not encoded the "to-be-remembered" stimulus effectively when it was initially shown, rather than forgetting what they had learned. Memory impairment did not increase with increasing delay and it is a decline in memory accuracy as a function of increasing delay (Sahakian et al., 1988) that is consistent with findings in patients with amnesia and human and non-human primates with lesions of the hippocampal formation, amygdala or medial temporal lobes (Sahakian et al., 1988; Joyce and Robbins, 1993; Owen et al., 1995; Elliott and Dolan, 1999; Chelonis et al., 2000).

Our findings add to the two extant studies in adults at risk for adult-onset schizophrenia or with early phase adult-onset schizophrenia (Wood et al., 2003; Mathes et al., 2005) and Luciana et al.'s (2005) developmental study of DMTS performance by suggesting that adolescents with undifferentiated schizophrenia have encoding but not retrieval deficits. Further, the sample studied addressed the potential neurodevelopmental confounds of gender, IQ and handedness.

Currently, it is thought that disruption to fronto-striatal dopaminergic neurocognitive systems interferes primarily with the encoding of stimuli and this can lead to memory impairments when those stimuli must be recognised after a delay. However, this impairment is independent of the length of time for which information must be held in memory. Specifically, activation of the caudate nucleus extending to the subgenual cingulate cortex (BA 24), the medial orbitofrontal cortex (BA 25 extending to 11) and the superior parietal cortex (BA 7) is seen during shorter delays on the DMTS task (Elliot and Dolan, 1999). In contrast, the published data (Sahakian et al., 1988; Lange et al., 1992; Robbins et al., 1997; Lawrence et al., 2000) suggest that delay-dependent memory impairments on the DMTS reflect disruption to cholinergically modulated neural circuits within the temporal lobe. Specifically, activation of the temporal pole (BA 21/38), medial temporal gyrus (BA 21), inferior temporal gyrus (BA 20), hippocampus and inferior frontal gyrus (BA 44/45) are associated with longer delays on the DMTS task (Elliot and Dolan, 1999) while the ability to encode stimuli is not disrupted. Our current results suggest only encoding fronto-striatal but not retrieval fronto-temporal neural systems are impaired in the medication naïve adolescents with undifferentiated schizophrenia. This finding is consistent with a developmental stage-independent dysfunction in schizophrenia. Importantly, these findings are consonant with the current conceptualization of schizophrenia as a neurodevelopmental disorder involving progressive gray and white matter changes from the parietal - temporal - frontal lobes (Thompson et al., 2001; Vidal et al., 2006).

In summary, medication naïve adolescents with undifferentiated schizophrenia were clearly only impaired in their encoding and accurately selecting the pattern of stimuli on the visuospatial memory task. Of clinical importance, adolescents with undifferentiated schizophrenia may demonstrate memory impairments when performing everyday and academically-related tasks. The current results suggest that such problems may be best dealt with by encouraging encoding of relevant information, rather than emphasising retrieval or recall strategies (that is, memory lists): Careful study of adolescent undifferentiated schizophrenia samples does detect deficits in a DMTS memory task, but these reflect attentional deficits rather than being specifically due to fronto-temporally mediated explicit memory system dysfunction.

The next study will address the nature of and association between visuospatial working memory and adolescent onset schizophrenia.

Study 2

Dysfunctional working memory systems subserved by the prefrontal cortex (PFC) (Goldman-Rakic and Selemon, 1997) may be associated with the core negative and disorganized symptoms of schizophrenia. To date, visuospatial working memory (VSWM) has been investigated because this construct is (1) largely non-verbal, (2) models of the relationship between VSWM and PFC are constrained by single neuronal firing rates in alert primates (Goldman –Rakic, 1987), studies of behaviour following focal PFC lesions in adult humans (Owen et al., 1993) and studies of patterns of regional cerebral blood flow in healthy humans performing VSWM tests (D'Esposito et al., 1995) and (3) the experimental paradigm used in these studies can be applied unchanged to the study of VSWM in children and adolescents (Barnett et al., 2001). Further the Cambridge Neuropsychological Test Automated Battery (CANTAB) (Owen et al., 1996) VSWM task has the additional benefit of allowing two key associated components of the dependent VSWM measure, 'between search error' (BSE) performance to be measured: (1) the ability to develop a systematic strategy during task performance (as reflected in the 'spatial strategy' measure) and (2) the ability to hold information 'on line' in a visuospatial scratchpad (Baddeley, 1986) (as reflected in the 'spatial span' measure) (Owen et al., 1990; Robbins, 1996; Panetlis et al., 1997). Hence, VSWM deficits, suggested by poor BSE performance, can be further analysed to see if this poor BSE performance relates to either or both of these components (Pantelis et al., 1997; Barnett et al., 2001).

This approach of parsing the construct of VSWM has been extended to the examination of putative underlying neural networks that may subserve the construct of VSWM and these key components. VSWM (as defined by 'BSE' or comparable measure performance) has been associated with activation of frontal-striatal-parietal neural networks, particularly the PFC and posterior parietal brain regions (Carlson et al., 1998; Braver et al., 1997; 2001). With respect to the PFC, VSWM is thought to 'rely' on the integrity of the dorsolateral prefrontal cortex (DLPFC) in non-human primates and human beings (Goldman-Rakic and Selemon, 1997; Cannon et al., 2005). Further, Owen et al. (1996) investigated VSWM in a PET study using tasks derived from 'BSE', 'spatial strategy' and 'spatial span' CANTAB measures. They reported that the 'organising, executing and monitoring' component, involving active monitoring and manipulation of spatial information (as reflected in 'spatial strategy'), may be associated with the mid-DLPFC (BA 46, 9), while the 'spatial span' component, involving a sequence of retained spatial moves in working memory, may be subserved by the ventrolateral prefrontal cortex (Brodmann Area (BA) 47).

To date, VSWM deficits (as defined by 'BSE' or comparable measure performance) have been shown in the acute and chronic phases of adult-onset schizophrenia (Pantelis et al., 1997; Wood et al., 2003) and those 'at-risk' for adult-onset schizophrenia (Glahn et al., 2003; Wood et al., 2003). Also, VSWM deficits are qualitatively similar but less severe in those with a broader phenotype of schizophrenia (Tsuang et al., 2002). Specifically, these VSWM deficits are associated with the 'spatial span' component in chronic adult-onset schizophrenia (Pantelis et al., 1997), acute adult-onset schizophrenia and those 'at-risk' for adult-onset schizophrenia (Wood et al., 2003), evident through between groups and correlational analyses. This study investigates whether VSWM deficits are (1) evident in adolescent-onset schizophrenia and (2) whether the relationships between components of VSWM are similar in adolescents to those reported in adults with schizophrenia.

Method

Participants

Nineteen right-handed male adolescents aged 12-17 years [14.64 (1.85) years] were identified with medication naïve, undifferentiated schizophrenia (DSM-IV, American Psychiatric Association, 1994) during their initial clinical evaluation before active treatment (Vance et al., 2006). This was defined through a semi-structured clinical interview (*Schedule for Affective Disorders and Schizophrenia – childhood version (K-SADS)*, Kaufman et al., 1997) with their parent(s) and with each adolescent [$\kappa > 0.80$] and by the clinician-completed *Positive and Negative Symptom Scale (PANSS)* (Kay et al., 1987): *Positive Scale* score of 67.11 (23.29) (percentile), a *Negative Scale* score of 79.53 (20.71) (percentile) and a *General Psychopathological Scale* score of 89.95 (21.30) (percentile). The undifferentiated schizophrenia group had a fullscale IQ of 109.10 (15.00) (*Wechsler Intelligence Scale for Children (WISC-3)* (Wechsler, 1991), with all fullscale IQs above 70 and a duration of illness of 12.45 (3.67) months. All the group were living in a family home and attending normal schools and none had overt neurological or endocrine disease or colour blindness. Twenty eight healthy male control participants were recruited through local schools, who did not meet criteria for any psychiatric, neurological or endocrine disorder, again defined through a semi-structured clinical interview *(K-SADS)*, Kaufman et al., 1997) with their parent(s) and with each adolescent and by the clinician-completed *PANSS* [(Kay et al.,1987): *Positive Scale* score of 2.11 (0.57) (percentile); $t(45) = 14.83$, $p < 0.0005$, a *Negative Scale* score of 1.71 (0.81) (percentile); $t(45) = 19.97$, $p < 0.0005$ and a *General Psychopathological Scale* score of 1.04 (0.19) (percentile); $t(45) = 22.20$, $p < 0.0005$] and who did not differ from the undifferentiated schizophrenia group in age [13.47 (1.77); $t(45)=1.58$, $p=0.12$] and fullscale IQ [105.89 (6.92); $t(45)= 0.98$, $p=0.33$].

Measures

Visuospatial working memory was assessed through measurement of performance on the Spatial Working Memory and Spatial Span tasks selected from the CANTAB (Owen et al., 1996). The computerised tests were presented on a high resolution IBM monitor with a touch sensitive screen. The Spatial Working Memory task is a self-ordered searching task that measures working memory for spatial stimuli and requires the subject to use mnemonic information to work towards a goal. Subjects are required to search through boxes that appear on the screen with the aim of finding the 'blue tokens' hidden inside. The key instruction was that once a token had been taken out of a box, that box would not be used again to hide a token. After two practice trials with two boxes, there were four test trials with each of two, three, four, six and eight boxes. Returning to an 'empty' box already opened and a token removed on a previous search constituted a 'forgetting' or 'Between Search' error (BSE). A Strategy score was calculated from subject's performance on the six and eight box levels, to reflect how often a searching sequence was initiated from the same box during a given trial. Higher Strategy scores represent low use of strategy (i.e., many sequences beginning with a different box in a given trial), and lower scores represent efficient use of strategy (i.e., many sequences starting with the same box in a given trial). The Spatial Span task is a computerised version of the Corsi block tapping test that assesses spatial short term memory capacity. This task measures the ability to remember a sequence of squares presented on the screen. After an incorrect attempt at choosing the squares in sequence, the next trial remains at the same difficulty level. The Spatial Span was calculated at the highest level at which the subject successfully remembered at least one sequence of boxes.

Statistical Analysis

Performance on the (1) BSE variable and (2) the Strategy and Spatial Span variables was compared between groups using respective (1) repeated measures and (2) one-way analysis of covariance (ANCOVA), co-varying for the effects of age and fullscale IQ, given the known sensitivity of these VSWM measures to these variables (Pantelis et al., 1997). To protect against experiment-wise error Type I error rates were set at $p<0.01$. To investigate the contribution of Spatial Span and Strategy to BSE, the intercorrelations between BSE and Span and between BSE and Strategy for all levels of difficulty were investigated for each group using Pearson product moment correlation coefficients.

Results

In the spatial working memory task, there was a significant effect of condition (number of boxes) [Wilks' $\lambda = 0.31$, $F(4,40) = 21.46$, $p < 0.0005$] and group [$F(1,43) = 9.54$, $p = 0.004$, partial $\eta^2 = 0.19$] with the undifferentiated schizophrenia group being associated with increased BSE, after controlling for age and fullscale IQ, only the latter having a significant independent association with BSE [F (1,43) = 25.82, $p < 0.0005$, partial $\eta^2 = 0.38$] (Figure 1). Also, there was a significant interaction between BSE and group [Wilks' $\lambda = 0.66$, F (4,40) = 4.99, $p = 0.002$], after controlling for age and fullscale IQ, again only the latter having a significant independent association with BSE [fullscale IQ: Wilks' $\lambda = 0.43$, F (4,40) = 12.99, $p < 0.0005$]. Neither Spatial Span [F (1,43) = 0.91, $p = 0.35$, partial $\eta^2 = 0.02$] (undifferentiated schizophrenia, 6.06 (1.21); control 6.39 (1.37)) nor Strategy [F (1,43) =0.42, $p = 0.52$, partial $\eta^2 = 0.01$] (undifferentiated schizophrenia, 31.99 (6.78); control 31.75 (3.97)) differed between the groups, after controlling for age and fullscale IQ, which had no independent association with either.

The pattern of intercorrelations between BSE, Spatial Span and Strategy was qualitatively different for the control [BSE: Spatial Span r = -0.11, $p = 0.59$; BSE: Strategy r = 0.31, $p = 0.12$] and undifferentiated schizophrenia groups [BSE: Spatial Span r = -0.26, $p = 0.32$; BSE: Strategy r = 0.51, $p = 0.04$], after controlling for age and fullscale IQ. For both groups, there was no correlation between Spatial Span and BSE. However there was a medium-large correlation between Strategy and BSE in the undifferentiated schizophrenia alone.

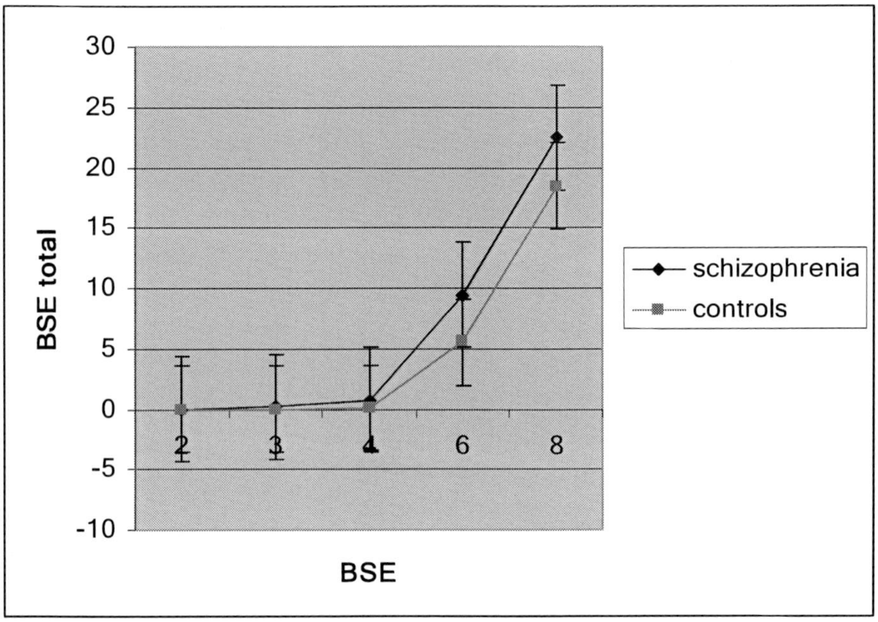

Figure 1. Between Search Errors (BSE - total score with standard error bars) at the 2,3,4,6 and 8 box levels of difficulty in the undifferentiated schizophrenia and healthy control groups.

Discussion

The adolescent-onset schizophrenia group is associated with increased negative and positive symptoms, consistent with previous studies of schizophrenia in this developmental phase (Schultz et al., 2000; Hollis et al., 2003). VSWM deficits (as defined by poor 'BSE' performance) are also evident, commensurate with Goldman-Rakic and Selemon's (1997) model and findings in adult-onset schizophrenia and the broader schizophrenia phenotype (Wood et al., 2003). Further, spatial span is spared in the adolescent-onset schizophrenia group in contrast to comparable data in adult-onset schizophrenia groups during 'at-risk', acute and chronic phases of illness (Pantelis et al., 1997; Wood et al., 2003), evident through between groups and correlational analyses. Spatial strategy is also spared in the adolescent-onset schizophrenia group consistent with comparable data in adult-onset schizophrenia groups (Wood et al., 2003), evident through between groups analysis. However, correlational analysis suggests that VSWM deficits (as defined by poor 'BSE' performance) are associated with spatial strategy in the adolescent-onset group unlike the adult-onset schizophrenia groups during 'at-risk', acute and chronic phases of illness (Pantelis et al., 1997; Wood et al., 2003).

These findings imply that frontal-striatal-parietal neural networks are dysfunctional in adolescent-onset schizophrenia, while mid-dorsolateral and ventrolateral PFC functions remain intact. In addition, the adolescent-onset schizophrenia group relied on spatial strategy rather than spatial span in their overall VSWM performance. In light of Wood et al.'s (2003) findings, this may suggest that the mid-dorsolateral PFC-linked fronto-parietal systems may be relatively more robust than the ventrolateral PFC fronto-parietal neural networks: there is emerging evidence that the ventrolateral PFC fronto-parietal neural networks (as reflected in the 'spatial span' component of VSWM) are less developed in adolescents compared to adults, whether schizophrenia is present or not (Saper et al., 2000; Luciana et al., 2005). As these fronto-parietal systems develop into adulthood, deficits in the ventrolateral PFC fronto-parietal neural networks (as reflected in the 'spatial span' component of VSWM) become apparent in adult-onset schizophrenia and those with the broader phenotype.

These possible progressive changes from one developmental phase to another are consistent with the current conceptualisation of schizophrenia as a neurodevelopmental disorder with progressive gray and white matter changes affecting the parietal through to frontal lobes (Thompson et al., 2001; Gogtay et al., 2004; Vidal et al., 2006). However, this study does not address the specificity of VSWM deficits for schizophrenia: future studies need to compare VSWM and its components performance across developmental phases in those with schizophrenia, those at risk of schizophrenia and those with the broader phenotype.

Integration and Implications of these Findings

The findings from both of these studies support the neurodevelopmental nature of schizophrenia, regardless of its age of onset. In particular, the findings are congruent with the known progressive maturation of gray and white matter neural networks in a caudal to rostral direction; that is from parietal through temporal to frontal regions. For instance, the determination of visuospatial memory encoding deficits in adolescents with undifferentiated schizophrenia is consistent with fronto-striatal-parietal neural network dysfunction that may arise from mainly parietal lobe region deficits. Visuospatial memory retrieval deficits, subserved by fronto-striatal-temporal neural networks, were not evident in the adolescents, unlike adults with schizophrenia. Hence, temporal lobe region-linked deficits may not yet be evident in the adolescents as they are in adults with schizophrenia. Similarly, visuospatial working memory deficits were evident in the adolescents with undifferentiated schizophrenia, implicating fronto-striatal-parietal neural network dysfunction while mid-dorsolateral and ventrolateral prefrontal cortical functions remained intact.

Future clinical research needs to [1] apply multiple cognitive neuroscience measures with well defined brain behaviour relationships that are able to parse visuospatial memory into encoding and retrieval components and working memory into capacitance and strategising components. Visuospatial rather than verbal memory and working memory measures remain preferable because they are relatively free of human language. Therefore, language learning and/or proficiency difficulties or disorders will not confound their interpretation. In addition, future clinical research needs to [2] apply functional magnetic resonance imaging (fMRI) paradigms that arise from these specific and targeted cognitive neuroscience measures; and investigate the associations of [1] and [2] with key candidate gene polymorphisms to systematically elucidate the neurodevelopmental pathophysiology of schizophrenia across key developmental stages such as adolescence and adulthood. Also, different subtypes of schizophrenia need to be systematically explored, specifically, disorganized, catatonic and paranoid forms of schizophrenia across key cultural and racial groups in which genetic influences may vary.

From a clinical perspective, these findings emphasize the importance of thorough clinical neuropsychological assessment of patients with schizophrenia. This assessment enables the inpatient and outpatient environments and treatment plan to be tailored to each given patient's executive functioning ability. Further, adolescents with schizophrenia require specific aid to encode information while adults require this help along with memory aids for their retrieval abilities. Possible future randomized controlled trials of stimulant medication, atomoxetine, and/or third line treatments for Attention Deficit Hyperactivity Disorder such as clonidine, imipramine or risperidone may be useful to best treat these memory encoding and working memory deficits.

References

Achenbach, T. M., 1991. *Manual for the Child Behavior Checklist* / 4-18 and 1991 Profile. University of Vermont, Burlington.

American Psychiatric Association, 1994. Diagnostic and Statistical Manual of Mental Disorders, fourth edition. *American Psychiatric Press,* Washington, DC.

Baddeley, A.D., 1986. *Working Memory.* Clarendon Press, Oxford.

Barnett, R., Vance, A.L.A., Maruff, P., Luk, S.L., Costin, J., Pantelis, C., 2001. Abnormal executive function in attention deficit hyperactivity disorder: The effect of stimulant medication and age on spatial working memory. *Psychological Medicine* 31, 1107-1115.

Barnett, R., Maruff, P., Vance, A., 2005. An investigation of visuospatial memory impairment in children with ADHD, combined type. *Psychological Medicine* 35, 1433-1443.

Bilder, R., Goldman, R., Robinson, D., 2000. Neuropsychology of first-episode schizophrenia: initial characterization and clinical correlates. *American Journal of Psychiatry* 157, 549-559.

Braver, T.S., Cohen, J.D., Nystrom, L.E., Jonides, J., Smith, E.E., Noll, D.C., 1997. A parametric study of prefrontal cortex involvement in human working memory. *Neuroimage* 5, 49-62.

Braver, T.S., Barch, D.M., Kelley, W.M., Buckner, R.L., Cohen, N.J., Miezen, F.M., Snyder, A.Z., Ollinger, J.M., Akbudak, E., Conturo, T.E., Petersen, S.E., 2001. Direct comparison of prefrontal cortex regions engaged by working and long-term memory tasks. *Neuroimage* 14, 48-59.

Brewer, W., Francey, S., Wood, S., 2005. Memory impairments identified in people at ultra-high risk for psychosis who later develop first-episode psychosis. *American Journal of Psychiatry* 162, 71-78.

Cannon, T.D., Glahn, D.C., Kim, J., Van Erp, T., Karlsgodt, K., Cohen, M.S., Nuechterlein, K.H., Bava, S., Shirinyan, D., 2005. Dorsolateral prefrontal cortex activity during maintenance and manipulation of information in working memory in patients with schizophrenia. *Archives of General Psychiatry* 62, 1071-1080.

Carlson, S., Martinkauppi, S., Rama, P., Salli, E., Korvenoja, A., Aronen, H.J., 1998. Distribution of cortical activation during visuospatial n-back tasks as revealed by functional magnetic resonance imaging. *Cerebral Cortex* 8, 743-752.

Chelonis, J.J., Daniels-Shaw, J. L., Blake, D. J., 2000. Developmental aspects of delayed matching-to-sample task performance in children. *Neurotoxicology Teratology* 22, 683-694.

D'Esposito, M., Detre, J. A., Alsop, D. C., Shin, R. K., Atlas, S., Grossman, M., 1995. The neural basis of the central executive system of working memory. *Nature,* 378, 279-281.

Devilbiss, D.M., Page, M.E., Waterhouse, B.D., 2006. Locus ceruleus regulates sensory encoding by neurons and networks in waking animals. *Journal of Neuroscience* 26, 9860-9872.

Elliot, R., Dolan, R.J., 1999. Differential neural responses during performance of matching and non-matching to sample tasks at two delay conditions. *Journal of Neuroscience* 19, 5066-5073.

Fleming, K., Goldberg, T.E., Binks, S., Randolph, C., Gold, J.M., Weinberger, D.R., 1997. Visuospatial working memory in patients with schizophrenia. *Biological Psychiatry* 41, 43-49.

Giedd, J.N., Lenane, M., Gochman, P., Evans, A., Rapoport, J.L., 2004. Comparison of progressive cortical gray matter loss in childhood-onset schizophrenia with that in childhood-onset atypical psychoses. *Archives of General Psychiatry* 61, 17-22.

Glahn, D.C., Therman, S., Manninen, M., Huttunen, M., Kaprio, J., Lonnqvist, J., Cannon, T.D., 2003. Spatial working memory as an endophenotype of schizophrenia. *Biological Psychiatry* 53, 624-626.

Gogtay, N., Sporn, A., Clasen, L.S., Nugent, T.F., Greenstein, D., Nicolson, R., Goldman-Rakic, P. S., 1987. Circuitry of the primate prefrontal cortex and the regulation of behaviour by representational memory. In F. Plum (Ed.), *Handbook of Physiology, The*

Nervous System, Higher functions of the Brain. Vol. V. American Physiological Society, Maryland, 373-417.

Goldman-Rakic, P.S., Selemon, L.D., 1997. Functional and anatomical aspects of prefrontal pathology in schizophrenia. *Schizophrenia Bulletin* 23, 437-458.

Hartman, M., Steketee, M., Silva, S., Lanning, K., McCann, H., 2002. Working memory and schizopohrenia: evidence for slowed encoding. *Schizophrenia Research* 59, 99-113.

Hollis, C., 2003. Developmental precursors of child- and adolescent-onset schizophrenia and affective psychoses: diagnostic specificity and continuity with symptom dimensions. *British Journal of Psychiatry* 182, 37-44.

Joyce, E.M., Robbins, T.W., 1991. Frontal lobe function in Korsakoff and non-Korsakoff alcoholics: planning and spatial working memory. *Neuropsychologica* 29, 709-723.

Kaufman, J., Birmaher, B., Brent, D., 1997. Schedule for Affective Disorders and Schizophrenia – present and lifetime version (K-SADS-PL): initial reliability and validity data. *Journal of the American Academy of Child and Adolescent Psychiatry* 36, 980-988.

Kay, S. R., Fiszbein, A., Opler, L.A., 1987. The Positive and Negative Syndrome Scale (PANSS) for schizophrenia. *Schizophrenia Bulletin* 13, 261-276.

Kravariti, E., Morris, R., Rabe-Hesketh, S., Murray, R.M., Frangou, S., 2003. The Maudsley Early-Onset Schizophrenia study: cognitive function in recent onset schizophrenia. *Schizophrenia Research* 61, 137-148.

Kravariti, E., Morris, R., Rabe-Hesketh, S., Murray, R.M., Frangou, S., 2003. The Maudsley Early-Onset Schizophrenia study: cognitive function in adolescent-onset schizophrenia. *Schizophrenia Research* 65, 95-103.

Lange, K. W., Robbins, T. W., Marsden, C. D.,1992. L-Dopa withdrawal in Parkinson's disease selectively impairs cognitive performance in tests sensitive to frontal dysfunction. *Psychopharmacology* 107, 394-404.

Lawrence, A.D., Watkins, L.H.A., Sahakian, B.J., 2000. Visual object and visuospatial cognition in Huntington's disease: implications for information processing in corticostriatal circuits. *Brain* 123, 1349-1364.

Leiderman, E., Strejilevich, S., 2004. Visuospatial deficits in schizophrenia: central executive and memory subsystem impairments. *Schizophrenia Research* 68, 217-223.

Luciana, M., Conklin, H.M., Hooper, C.J., Yarger, R.S., 2005. The development of nonverbal working memory and executive control processes in adolescents. *Child Development* 76, 697-712.

Maruff, P., Tyler, P., Burt, T.,1996. Cognitive deficits in Machado-Joseph Disease. *Annals of Neurology* 40, 421-427.

Mathes, B., Wood, S.J., Proffitt, T.M., 2005. Early processing deficits in object working memory in first episode schizophreniform psychosis and established schizophrenia. *Psychological Medicine* 35, 1053-1062.

Owen, A.M., Downes, J.J., Sahakian, B.J., Polkey, C.E., Robbins, T.W., 1990. Planning and spatial working memory following frontal lesions in man. *Neuropsychologia* 28, 1021-1034.

Owen, A. M., Roberts, A. C., Hodges, J. R., Summers, B. A., Polkey, C. E., Robbins, T. W., 1993. Contrasting mechanisms of attentional set-shiftng in patients with frontal lobe damage or Parkinson's Disease. *Brain,* 116, 1159-1175.

Owen, A. M., Sahakian, B. J., Semple, J., 1995. Visuo-spatial short-term recognition memory and learning after temporal lobe excisions, frontal lobe excisions or amygdalo-hippocampectomy in man. *Neuropsychologia* 33, 1-24.

Owen, A.M., Evans, A.C., Petrides, M., 1996. Evidence for a two-stage model of spatial working memory processing within the lateral frontal cortex: a positron emission tomography study. *Cerebral Cortex* 6, 31-38.

Pantelis, C., Barnes, T.R.E., Nelson, H.E., Tanner, S., Weatherley, L., Owen, A.M., Robbins, T.W., 1997. Frontal-striatal cognitive deficits in patients with chronic schizophrenia. *Brain* 120, 1823-1843.

Pantelis, C., Stuart, G., Hazel, N., 2001. Spatial working memory deficits in schizophrenia: relationship with tardive dyskinesia and negative symptoms. *American Journal of Psychiatry* 158, 1276-1285.

Paule, M.G., Bushnell, P. J., Maurissen, J. P. J., 1998. Symposium Overview: The use of delayed matching-to-sample procedures in studies of short-term memory in animals and humans. *Neurotoxicology Teratology* 20, 493-502.

Rhinewine, J., Lencz, T., Thaden, E.P., 2005. Neurocognitive profile in adolescents with early onset schizophrenia: clinical correlates. *Biological Psychiatry* 58, 705-712.

Robbins, T.W., 1996. Dissociating executive functions of the prefrontal cortex. *Philosophical Transactions of the Royal Society of London B Biological Sciences* 351, 1463-1470.

Robbins, T .W., Semple, J., Kumar, R., 1997. Effects of scopolamine on delayed matching to sample and paired associates of visual memory and learning in human subjects: comparison with diazepam and implications for dementia. *Psychopharmacology* 134, 95-106.

Rund, B.R., Melle, I., Friis, S., Larson, T.K., Midboe, L.J., Opjordsmeon, S., Simonsen, E., Vaglum, P., McGlashan, T., 2004. Neurocognitive dysfunction in first-episode psychosis: correlates with symptoms, premorbid adjustment and duration of untreated psychosis. *American Journal of Psychiatry* 161, 466-472.

Sahakian, B. J., Morris, R. G., Evenden, J. L., 1988. A comparative study of visuospatial memory and learning in Alzheimer-type dementia and Parkinson's disease. *Brain* 111, 695-718.

Saper, C.B., Iverson, S., Frackowiak, R., 2000. Integration of sensory and motor function: the association areas of the cerebral cortex and the cognitive capabilities of the human brain. In: Kandel, E.R., Schwartz, J.H., Jessell, T.M. (Eds.), *Principles of Neural Science.* McGraw Hill, New York, pp. 349-380.

Schultz, S.K., Ho, B.C., Andreasen, N.C., 2000. Clinical features characterising young-onset and intermediate-onset schizophrenia. *Journal of Neuropsychiatry and Clinical Neurosciences* 12, 502-505.

Smith, C., Park, S., Cornblatt, B., 2006. Spatial working memory deficits in adolescents at clinical high risk for schizophrenia. *Schizophrenia Research* 81, 211-215.

Tan, H., Choo, W., Fones, C., Chee, M., 2005. fMRI study of maintenance and manipulation processes within working memory in first-episode schizophrenia. *American Journal of Psychiatry* 162, 1849-1858.

Tabachnick, B. G., Fidell, L. S., 2001. *Using Multivariate Statistics*, fourth edition. Allyn and Bacon, Boston.

Thompson, P.M., Vidal, C., Giedd, J.N., Gochman, P., Blumenthal, J., Nicolson, R, Toga, A.W., Rapoport, J.L., 2001. Mapping adolescent brain change reveals dynamic wave of accelerated gray matter loss in very early-onset schizophrenia. *Proceedings of the National Academy of Sciences,* USA 98, 11650-11655.

Tsuang, M.T., Stone, W.S., Tarbox, S.I., Faraone, S.V., 2002. An integration of schizophrenia with schizotypy: identification of schizotaxia and implications for research on treatment and prevention. *Schizophrenia Bulletin* 54, 169-175.

Vance, A., Hall, N., Bellgrove, M., Casey, M., Karsz, F., Maruff, P., 2006. Visuospatial working memory deficits in adolescent onset schizophrenia. *Schizophrenia Research* 87: 223-227.

Vance, A., Hall, N., Casey, M., Karsz, F., Bellgrove, M., 2007. Visuospatial memory deficits in adolescent onset schizophrenia. *Schizophrenia Research* 93; 345-349.

Vidal, C., Rapoport, J.L., Hayashi, K.M., Geaga, J.A., Sui, Y., McLemore, L.E., Alaghband, Y., Giedd, J.N., Gochman, P., Blumenthal, J., Gogtay, N., Nicolson, R., Toga, A.W., Thompson, P.M., 2006. Dynamically spreading frontal and cingulated deficits mapped in adolescents with schizophrenia. *Archives of General Psychiatry* 63, 25-34.

Wechsler, D., 1991. *Wechsler Intelligence Scale for Children,* third edition. The Psychological Co-operation, Texas.

Wood, S.J., Pantelis, C., Proffitt, T., Phillips, L.J., Stuart, G.W., Buchanan, J.A., Mahoney, K., Brewer, W., Smith, D.J., McGorry, P.D., 2003. Spatial working memory ability is a marker of risk-for-psychosis. *Psychological Medicine* 33, 1239-1247.

Zakzanis, K.K., 2001. Statistics to tell the truth, the whole truth and nothing but the truth: formulae, illustrative numerical examples, and heuristic interpretation of effect size analyses for neuropsychological researchers. *Archives of Clinical Neuropsychology* 16, 653-667.

In: Adolescent Schizophrenia
Editors: J. T. Nillinghouse and R. P. Trotman

ISBN: 978-1-60692-370-2

Chapter III

Psychotic Symptoms in Children and Adolescents

Michelle Harley[1,2], Aileen Murtagh[2], Ian Kelleher[1] and Mary Cannon[1]

[1]Department of Psychiatry, Royal College of Surgeons in Ireland, Dublin, Ireland
[2]Department of Child and Adolescent Psychiatry, Mater Misericordiae Hospital, Dublin, Ireland
[2]Department of Child and Adolescent Psychiatry, National Children's Hospital, Tallaght, Dublin, Ireland

Abstract

Recent studies suggest that psychosis exists along a continuum in the general population, rather than as an all-or-none phenomenon. This is supported by the finding that the prevalence of psychotic symptoms in the general population far exceeds the prevalence of psychotic disorders. Only 1% of the overall population will develop schizophrenia during their lifetime whereas international epidemiological research suggests that between 5% and 38% of the adult general population may experience at least one psychotic symptom in their lives, with rates of 2.1% to 58.9 % reported for child and adolescent populations. The significance of psychotic symptoms in children and adolescents is not as yet fully established: they have been found to be associated with a variety of psychiatric disorders in this age group, in particular depression and anxiety, and social factors including childhood abuse. There is emerging evidence that psychotic symptoms in childhood and adolescence may be risk markers for psychotic illness in adulthood. Poulton et al (1999) [1] found that self-reported psychotic symptoms at age 11 years predicted a very high risk of a schizophrenia spectrum disorder at age 26 years. Therefore, adolescents who report psychotic symptoms could be conceptualised as a 'high risk' group for schizophrenia. This paradigm may prove valuable in exploring early risk factors for psychosis-vulnerability and in predicting psychotic outcomes.

Introduction

Recent research suggests that psychotic symptoms in both clinical and community samples of children and adolescents are relatively common [1-3] and exist on a continuum in the population in children and adolescents as well as in adults [4]. These symptoms can exist in persons with a range of non-psychotic psychiatric illnesses and also in healthy individuals of all ages who are functioning well [3, 4]. Despite these findings, even in clinical settings, psychotic symptoms are not routinely asked about in children and adolescents. The narrow definition of psychotic symptoms according to classical phenomenology includes delusions or prominent hallucinations with absence of insight into their pathological nature, however more recent studies have begun to look at wider definitions of psychotic symptoms to include terms such as “attenuated”, “subthreshold” or “subclinical” psychotic symptoms, or “psychotic like experiences” [3, 5-7].

Much of the research into schizophrenia over the past decade has focussed on the schizophrenic “prodrome”, looking at “high risk” and “ultra high risk” groups and factors predicting progression to full-blown psychotic illness in these groups [8, 9]. Psychotic symptoms constitute an important part of the “prodromal” phase of psychiatric illness and prodromal symptoms in community samples across the lifespan. To meet ultra high risk criteria, psychotic symptoms must be of sufficient severity and frequency and must have begun or worsened within the last year [10] however isolated psychotic symptoms can occur long before the prodromal phase of schizophrenia, and some studies suggest that they may be an early risk factor for later psychotic illness [1, 11] although the prognostic significance of their presence in non-psychotic children and adolescents is not yet clear.

How Common Are Psychotic Symptoms?

Prevalence in Adult Populations

Prevalence figures for psychotic symptoms in adults range from 5% to 38% in community samples [5, 12-23]. In the US National Household Survey on Drug Abuse [5], 5.1% of 38132 adults reported one or more psychotic like experiences in the past year. The Epidemiological Catchment Area study in the U.S. reported that 10.2% of males and 14.9% of females had had more than one lifetime experience of non-organic hallucinations (sample size 18572) [24]. In the Australian National Survey of Mental Health and Wellbeing, 11.7% of 10641 adults reported one or more lifetime delusional experience [25]. The highest rate of psychotic symptoms was reported in the Canadian Ohayon study, in which 38.7% of a sample of 13057 aged over 15 years reported current hallucinatory experiences [26]. For review of studies of the prevalence of psychotic symptoms in adult populations, see Laurens et al. [3].

Prevalence in Child and Adolescent Populations

General Population Samples

Fewer studies have been carried out examining the prevalence of psychotic symptoms in child and adolescent than in adult samples. As part of the Dunedin Multidisciplinary Health and Development study, a longitudinal study of the health and development of a birth cohort in New Zealand, 789 children were interviewed by a child and adolescent psychiatrist at age 11 years using the Diagnostic Interview Schedule for children. 14.7% of the sample endorsed at least one psychotic symptom at age 11 years, including 8% who reported at least sometimes experiencing hallucinatory phenomena [1, 27]. A 2004 Japanese study screened a community sample of 761 children aged 11 – 12 years recruited from schools using a questionnaire about auditory and visual hallucinatory experiences, and found that 21% of the sample had experienced hallucinations at some time in their lives [2]. Dhossche et al (2002) examined 914 adolescents aged 11-18 years participating in an ongoing longitudinal study and reported that hallucinations had been experienced by 6% of adolescents and 3% of young adults at baseline [28]. An Australian study found that 51% of 657 high school students endorsed often or occasional magical ideation, 45.6% unusual perceptual experiences and 25.2% markedly peculiar behaviour [29]. Laurens et al (2007) screened a community sample of 567 children aged 9 to 12 years for psychotic symptoms, emotional behavioural difficulties and developmental delay using questionnaires [3]. Follow up interviews were carried out by a child psychiatrist on 13% of the sample, randomly selected, of whom 58.9% reported "certain" experience of at least one psychotic symptom. Follow up interviews demonstrated moderate agreement between child and clinician ratings of "psychotic-like experiences".

In summary, rates of psychotic symptoms in community child and adolescent samples across the small number of studies carried out to date range from 6% to 58.9%. This wide variation is likely to be partly the result of differing methodology used to identify psychotic symptoms, as there is no standard developmentally appropriate screening instrument for psychotic symptoms in children and adolescents. Also, some studies only examined hallucinatory experiences and not other psychotic symptoms, while some studies looked at current psychotic symptoms and others enquired about lifetime experience of symptoms.

Clinical Child and Adolescent Samples

Early studies investigating rates of psychotic symptoms in children and adolescents looked at clinical samples and found a wide range of results: in 1962, Eisenberg reported that 0.4% of 14000 outpatient children reported hallucinations [30]; in 1962 Jaffe et al reported a rate as high as 63% in a state hospital population [31], and in 1972 Edgell & Kolvin reported a rate of 5% in an inpatient population aged 5-15 years [32]. In a 1975 study, Simonds found that 2.3% of children admitted to an inpatient unit over a 3 year period reported hallucinations [33]. Elena Garralda (1984) reported an estimated incidence of hallucinations in clinical populations as 1.1% based on a retrospective chart review of children seen at the Maudesley Hospital over a 12 year period [34].

A more recent small US study carried out in 1997 in a sample of 38 adolescents attending a residential centre and day treatment program found that 33% of participants reported having experienced auditory hallucinations, and 24% had delusional ideation [35]. Chambers et al

(1982) found that 38% of a sample of 58 children aged 6 to 12 years with major depressive disorders reported hallucinations, but less than 7% had delusions [36]. Famularo et al (1992) reported an incidence of 9% for hallucinations among a population of maltreated children [37]. In a similar population, 29% of 96 homeless adolescents were found to have psychotic symptoms in a study by Mundy et al (1990) [38]. In summary, sample prevalences from clinical or at risk groups in published studies range from 0.4% to 63%.

Why Are we Interested in Psychotic Symptoms?

Family history is currently The earliest predictor currently of future schizophreniform disorder, with a 6 to 10 fold reported increase in risk in probands who have a first-degree relative who suffers from bipolar disorder or schizophrenia [39] however the majority (63%) of people who go on to develop schizophrenia do not have an affected relative [40]. In the Dunedin birth cohort study, children who reported psychotic symptoms at age 11 were found to be at a much higher risk of later schizophreniform disorder than those who did not [1]. This finding suggests that children who report psychotic symptoms can be conceptualised as a "high risk" group for adult clinical psychosis, providing a unique paradigm for exploring early risk factors for psychosis vulnerability. The findings from the Dunedin study have not yet been replicated, however in support of this hypothesis research on the correlates of psychotic symptoms has shown remarkably similar findings to research specifically on those with clinical psychotic illnesses in adult populations, including associations with single marital status, blunting of affect, lower quality of life, lower age, lower level of education, depressive symptoms, and urbanicity [17, 41]and also with cannabis dependence, alcohol dependence, recent stressful life events, lower intellectual ability, neurotic symptoms and victimisation [20].

Factors Associated with Psychotic Symptoms in Childhood

Psychiatric Associations

Psychotic symptoms in childhood and adolescence have been linked to several psychiatric disorders other than schizophrenia. Significant levels of depression and/or anxiety have repeatedly been reported in children with psychotic symptoms [33, 34, 36, 42-49]. Other reported mental health associations include conduct disorder [48] and substance use, including cannabis use, in adolescence [50]. Dissociative experiences and Post Traumatic Stress Disorder (PTSD) related to physical and sexual abuse have also been reported to be associated with psychotic symptoms in child and adolescent samples [37, 51].

Psychosocial Factors

A number of authors have reported increased rates of childhood abuse [37, 52-54] and increased rates of exposure to domestic violence [47, 54] among children and adolescents who describe psychotic symptoms - a finding that mirrors the clinical picture of psychosis in adults [55, 56]. Burke et al (1985) however found no significant differences between hallucinating and non-hallucinating groups for recent or past history of physical or sexual abuse in a retrospective study of 40 child psychiatry inpatients [57]. A strong association has been reported between psychotic symptoms in childhood and bully/victim status (that is, a child who has been identified as both a perpetrator and a victim of bullying) [54]. This finding has not been reported among clinical cohorts; however, research interest in "bully/victims" is a recent development. Bully/victims (as opposed to "pure" victims) tend to develop more pervasive and more severe psychological and behavioural outcomes [58]. They also tend to come from homes where the parents are less involved and more likely to be hostile and rejecting [59], a finding that fits well with the associations of abuse and neglect reported in adolescent populations with subclinical manifestations of psychosis [54] and in adult populations with psychotic disorders [55, 56].

Other social factors associated with psychotic symptoms in children and adolescents include a background of family break up, psychiatric illness and/or alcohol abuse [47]. Higher rates of clinical psychosis among Black/Caribbean ethnic groups have reported in adults [60, 61] and also in adolescent populations [62, 63]. This finding is mirrored by the reports that psychotic symptoms are more common in Black/Caribbean-British than in the White-British population in both adult [18], and child [63] populations. Patino et al (2005) reported the related finding that psychotic symptoms in their sample of children and adolescents were twice as frequent in those with a history of migration, and additionally that these symptoms were four times more frequent in those with a history of both migration and family dysfunction [64].

Outcome of Psychotic Symptoms in Childhood

Follow up studies of non-psychotic children who report psychotic symptoms show that there appears to be a high rate of discontinuation when they are followed up even for short periods of several months [43, 48, 65]. This is similar to findings in adult populations [66]. However, compared with the rest of the population, there are increased rates of adult mental illness among children and adolescents reporting such symptoms [1, 28, 67]. The prognostic significance of psychotic symptoms in non-psychotic children and adolescents is unclear as the results of the few published follow up studies are conflicting. Elena Garralda, in the early 1980s, prospectively followed a cohort of 20 children with conduct and emotional disorders and found that auditory hallucinations were not associated with later psychiatric disorder (psychotic disorder and depressive disorder) [68]. Other studies have reached a different conclusion however. Several years later, Del Beccaro et al (1988) found that hallucinations in an inpatient psychiatric sample of 25 non-psychotic children carried a poor prognosis, with 20% having had an episode of acute psychosis at follow up 4 years later, and another 28%

believed to exhibit atypical psychoses. Children who hallucinated in this sample exhibited more behavioural disturbance than inpatients who did not [11]. Escher et al (2002) followed up a group of 80 children aged 8 – 19 years with auditory hallucinations and found a cumulative discontinuation rate of 60%. In this study, the authors noted that hallucinations were more likely to persist if they were severe and frequent or if they were associated with anxiety and depression [65]. In contrast to these findings, Askenazy et al (2007) reported results of a study following up 90 children aged 5 to 12 years for a period of one year. The authors found that 18% (16/90) reported auditory hallucinations at baseline. They differentiated between two groups of children: 53% of children, all of whom had anxiety disorders, had fully recovered from hallucinations at one year whereas another 30%, all of whom had a conduct disorder, showed persistence of these symptoms over a 12 month period. No child in the study was diagnosed with schizophrenia [48].

In the Dunedin study, a large New Zealand birth cohort were interviewed at age 11 years using the Diagnostic Interview Schedule for Children, and again at age 26 years. This study found that children who had reported psychotic symptoms at age 11 years were 16 times more likely to have developed a schizophreniform illness by age 26. They were also, to a lesser extent, more likely to have developed an anxiety disorder but not a depressive disorder [1]. Dhossche et al [28] assessed a community sample of 914 adolescents aged 11 to 18 using the Youth Self-Report Questionnaire [69], and followed them up 8 years later using a semi-structured interview: the Composite International Diagnostic interview [70]. 783/914 adolescents were interviewed at follow up, and self-reported hallucinations were found to be associated with concurrent non-psychotic psychiatric problems in both age groups (no participant was diagnosed with a psychotic disorder). Those who reported auditory but not visual hallucinations had higher rates of depressive disorders and substance use disorders, but not psychotic disorders, compared to controls.

Comparing the results of longitudinal studies on the outcomes associated with psychotic symptoms in children and adolescents reveals a marked variability in outcomes between studies. This may be in part due to selection bias as some of these studies were of clinical samples selected using differing methodology, and some were of community samples. As Schreier commented in his 1999 paper on hallucinations in non-psychotic children "our knowledge of the nature and consequences of hallucinations in childhood is biased by the populations in which they have been studied" [71]. As with studies of prevalence, lack of agreement between studies is likely to be partly the result of varying methodology, as there is no standard screening instrument for psychotic symptoms in children and adolescents.

An important question that has not yet been answered is whether specific psychotic symptoms carry more prognostic significance than others, and if so which ones and for what disorders? For example, hearing a phone ringing or hearing one's name being called is a frequent symptom in normal populations and may be almost a "normal" phenomenon. Musical hallucinations have been found to be associated with Obsessive Compulsive Disorder [72]. Some psychotic symptoms may be more likely to be associated with later psychotic disorders, but this will need to be established through longitudinal studies of child and adolescent populations screening for psychotic symptoms at baseline.

How Might Psychotic Symptoms Lead to Psychosis?

If there is an increased risk of later psychotic disorder associated with the presence of psychotic symptoms in childhood, then the question arises as to the pathway by which these symptoms might lead to clinical psychosis. Cougnard et al [73] have proposed the hypothesis that "common, non-clinical developmental expression of psychosis may become abnormally persistent when synergistically combined with developmental exposures that may impact on behavioural and neurotransmitter sensitization such as cannabis, trauma and urbanicity" and tested this in two adult general population samples: the Dutch Mental Health Survey and Incidence Study (NEMESIS) [74, 75], and a German study: The Early Developmental Stages of Psychopathology (EDSP) [76]. The authors concluded that environmental risks for psychosis act additively, and that the level of environmental risk combines synergistically with non-clinical psychotic symptoms to cause abnormal persistence. This has not yet been shown for child and adolescent populations, but a similar interaction may exist. Further evidence for an interaction between developmental exposures in the causation of psychosis comes from a recent study by Houston et al (2007), who re-examined data from the National Comorbidity Survey. They reported no significant association between a diagnosis of psychosis in adulthood and either early cannabis use or childhood sexual abuse, however they found a significant effect in those who had been the victims of sexual trauma in childhood and who had also used cannabis before the age of 16 years [77].

Can we Screen for Psychotic Symptoms?

One difficulty that arises when assessing psychotic symptoms in children is particular to this age group; the ability to differentiate imagination from reality depends on the developmental stage of the child, so that in younger children it can be difficult to determine what constitutes a psychotic symptom [32]. In addition, younger children have immature language and cognitive development and may find it difficult to describe their symptoms accurately. Instruments such as the Psychosis screening questionnaire [78] are available for use in adult populations however no instruments for screening for psychotic symptoms in child populations using developmentally appropriate questions are available as yet. Detailed instruments exist for assessing psychotic symptoms in depth once screening has been carried out, such as the Structured Interview for Prodromal Syndromes (SIPS) [10]. In some studies where a screening questionnaire was required, authors have designed and used their own questionnaire, or extracted questions from an established interview instrument, for example in the Dunedin study [1] five questions from the psychosis section of the Diagnostic Interview Schedule for Children [79] were used to screen for psychotic symptoms, and these same questions were used again by Laurens et al to screen a community sample of children [3]. General questionnaires such as the Youth Self Report [69] have also been used in some studies [28]. The PRIME Clinic in the USA has developed a 12-item psychosis-specific self-report screening questionnaire [80].

The outcome of studies of studies aiming to detect psychotic symptoms in young people may be influenced by the method of assessment used, so that this requires careful consideration. Children and adolescents may be more comfortable reporting psychotic symptoms on self-report questionnaires, than during clinical interviews. Laurens et al found that higher rates of psychotic symptoms were reported by children on self-report questionnaires than in previous studies which had used interview techniques [3]. It is also important that children understand the questions asked, and that under or over-reporting of psychotic symptoms doesn't occur through misinterpretation of questions. Age, cognitive and language ability may all influence content and expression of symptoms.

Ethical Issues

Clearly there is value in identifying young people at risk of psychosis in order to monitor their mental health and possibly intervene early to prevent or delay the onset of frank psychosis. It is not yet established how strong a risk factor is constituted by psychotic symptoms without other prodromal symptoms in children and adolescents, nor what outcomes these symptoms are a risk factor for. Screening for psychotic symptoms in this population in order to identify those with an increased vulnerability to psychosis raises a number of ethical questions, not least how to disclose this information to those who are identified as being at risk, the possibility of stigma, and the potential effects on family dynamics. Closely related to these ethical considerations is the question of whether or not useful intervention is possible in this group of children and adolescents at risk of psychosis.

Can we Treat Isolated Psychotic Symptoms in Children and Adolescents?

Recent research has focused on interventions in the prodromal phase of illness in those thought to be at ultra-high risk of incipient psychosis in late adolescence or early adulthood. The efficacy of cognitive therapy [81-83], olanzapine [84, 85] and a combination of risperidone and cognitive behavioural therapy [86] have been evaluated in this group. Although some positive results have been reported, the evidence-base is weak and further research is needed [87]. There is a paucity of research on interventions for psychotic symptoms at an even earlier stage, before criteria for the ultra-high risk state are met. For young people who are help-seeking and present to child and adolescent mental health services due to their psychotic and/or other symptoms, monitoring over time for persistence of and change in psychotic symptoms, functional decline and comorbid psychopathology and assessment of their coping strategies is appropriate. It is postulated that transitions over the psychosis continuum are in part driven by emotional, cognitive and behavioural responses to psychotic experiences. Delusional interpretation, negative emotional states and/or a symptomatic coping style carry an increased risk for the development of a psychotic disorder [88]. Family interventions, social skills training and cognitive behavioural therapy may be appropriate interventions for a child presenting with psychotic symptoms in the absence of a diagnosis of a psychotic disorder, depending on presentation and clinical need.

Conclusion

In summary, psychotic symptoms in children and adolescents are far more common than previously thought, however their prognostic significance is not yet clear. They may be a risk factor for later psychotic illness, or a marker for general psychopathology. Studies are lacking in this area, in particular large-scale epidemiological studies of the prevalence of these symptoms with follow up in prospective cohort studies from childhood to adulthood to determine outcomes associated with these symptoms and to identify the individual differences that demarcate those who become clinically psychotic from those who remain well. A well-validated developmentally appropriate screening questionnaire for the identification of psychotic symptoms in children and adolescents would be a useful tool to further research in this area. Psychotic symptoms in children and adolescents have a number of psychiatric and psychosocial correlates, some of which mirror the correlates of psychotic illness in adults and adolescents.

While most research in this area has focused on psychotic symptoms in adults, a literature is beginning to emerge on children and adolescents with psychotic symptoms suggesting that they represent a unique and valuable population for examining why, given that these symptoms are relatively common in the general population, some individuals proceed to full blown psychosis while most do not. This information could prove highly valuable in furthering our understanding of the aetiology of clinical psychosis, as well as providing information on specific and sensitive risk factors predictive of clinical conversion to psychosis. Given the potential benefits of early intervention in psychosis, targeting individuals at the earliest stage possible could be extremely beneficial and could even lead to primary prevention in psychiatry.

References

[1] Poulton, R., et al., Children's self-reported psychotic symptoms and adult schizophreniform disorder: a 15-year longitudinal study. *Arch Gen Psychiatry,* 2000. 57(11): p. 1053-8.

[2] Yoshizumi, T., et al., Hallucinatory experiences in a community sample of Japanese children. *J Am Acad Child Adolesc Psychiatry,* 2004. 43(8): p. 1030-6.

[3] Laurens, K.R., et al., Community screening for psychotic-like experiences and other putative antecedents of schizophrenia in children aged 9-12 years. *Schizophr Res,* 2007. 90(1-3): p. 130-46.

[4] Verdoux, H. and J. van Os, Psychotic symptoms in non-clinical populations and the continuum of psychosis. *Schizophr Res,* 2002. 54(1-2): p. 59-65.

[5] Mojtabai, R., Psychotic-like experiences and interpersonal violence in the general population. *Soc Psychiatry Psychiatr Epidemiol,* 2006. 41(3): p. 183-90.

[6] Loewy, R.L., J.K. Johnson, and T.D. Cannon, Self-report of attenuated psychotic experiences in a college population. *Schizophr Res,* 2007. 93(1-3): p. 144-51.

[7] Rossler, W., et al., Psychotic experiences in the general population: a twenty-year prospective community study. *Schizophr Res,* 2007. 92(1-3): p. 1-14.

[8] Yung, A.R. and P.D. McGorry, Prediction of psychosis: setting the stage. *Br J Psychiatry Suppl,* 2007. 51: p. s1-8.

[9] Cannon, T.D., et al., Prediction of psychosis in youth at high clinical risk: a multisite longitudinal study in North America. *Arch Gen Psychiatry,* 2008. 65(1): p. 28-37.

[10] Miller, T.J., et al., Symptom assessment in schizophrenic prodromal states. *Psychiatr Q,* 1999. 70(4): p. 273-87.

[11] Del Beccaro, M.A., P. Burke, and E. McCauley, Hallucinations in children: a follow-up study. *J Am Acad Child Adolesc Psychiatry,* 1988. 27(4): p. 462-5.

[12] Ross, C.A., S. Joshi, and R. Currie, Dissociative experiences in the general population. *Am J Psychiatry,* 1990. 147(11): p. 1547-52.

[13] Eaton, W.W., et al., Screening for psychosis in the general population with a self-report interview. *J Nerv Ment Dis,* 1991. 179(11): p. 689-93.

[14] Kendler, K.S., et al., Lifetime prevalence, demographic risk factors, and diagnostic validity of nonaffective psychosis as assessed in a US community sample. The National Comorbidity Survey. *Arch Gen Psychiatry,* 1996. 53(11): p. 1022-31.

[15] Verdoux, H., et al., A survey of delusional ideation in primary-care patients. *Psychol Med,* 1998. 28(1): p. 127-34.

[16] Peters, E.R., S.A. Joseph, and P.A. Garety, Measurement of delusional ideation in the normal population: introducing the PDI (Peters et al. Delusions Inventory). *Schizophr Bull,* 1999. 25(3): p. 553-76.

[17] van Os, J., et al., Strauss (1969) revisited: a psychosis continuum in the general population? *Schizophr Res,* 2000. 45(1-2): p. 11-20.

[18] Johns, L.C., et al., Occurrence of hallucinatory experiences in a community sample and ethnic variations. *Br J Psychiatry,* 2002. 180: p. 174-8.

[19] Olfson, M., et al., Psychotic symptoms in an urban general medicine practice. *Am J Psychiatry,* 2002. 159(8): p. 1412-9.

[20] Johns, L.C., et al., Prevalence and correlates of self-reported psychotic symptoms in the British population. *Br J Psychiatry,* 2004. 185: p. 298-305.

[21] King, M., et al., Psychotic symptoms in the general population of England--a comparison of ethnic groups (The EMPIRIC study). *Soc Psychiatry Psychiatr Epidemiol,* 2005. 40(5): p. 375-81.

[22] Vega, W.A., et al., Putative psychotic symptoms in the Mexican American population: prevalence and co-occurrence with psychiatric disorders. *J Nerv Ment Dis,* 2006. 194(7): p. 471-7.

[23] Wiles, N.J., et al., Self-reported psychotic symptoms in the general population: results from the longitudinal study of the British National Psychiatric Morbidity Survey. *Br J Psychiatry,* 2006. 188: p. 519-26.

[24] Tien, A.Y., Distributions of hallucinations in the population. *Soc Psychiatry Psychiatr Epidemiol,* 1991. 26(6): p. 287-92.

[25] Scott, J., et al., Psychotic-like experiences in the general community: the correlates of CIDI psychosis screen items in an Australian sample. *Psychol Med,* 2006. 36(2): p. 231-8.

[26] Ohayon, M.M., Prevalence of hallucinations and their pathological associations in the general population. *Psychiatry Res,* 2000. 97(2-3): p. 153-64.

[27] McGee, R., S. Williams, and R. Poulton, Hallucinations in nonpsychotic children. *J Am Acad Child Adolesc Psychiatry,* 2000. 39(1): p. 12-3.

[28] Dhossche, D., et al., Diagnostic outcome of self-reported hallucinations in a community sample of adolescents. *Psychol Med,* 2002. 32(4): p. 619-27.

[29] McGorry, P.D., et al., The prevalence of prodromal features of schizophrenia in adolescence: a preliminary survey. *Acta Psychiatr Scand,* 1995. 92(4): p. 241-9.

[30] L, E., Hallucinations in children. *Hallucinations,* ed. L.J.W.N. York. 1962: Grune & Stratton.

[31] Jaffe, S.L., Hallucinations in children at a state hospital. *Psychiatr Q,* 1966. 40(1): p. 88-95.

[32] Edgell HG, K.I., Childhood hallucinations. *J. Child Psychol. Psychiatry,* 1972(13): p. 279 - 287.

[33] Simonds, J.F., Hallucinations in Nonpsychotic Children and Adolescents. *Journal of Youth and Adolescence,* 1975. 4(2): p. 11.

[34] Garralda, M.E., Hallucinations in children with conduct and emotional disorders: I. The clinical phenomena. *Psychol Med,* 1984. 14(3): p. 589-96.

[35] Altman, H., M. Collins, and P. Mundy, Subclinical hallucinations and delusions in nonpsychotic adolescents. *J Child Psychol Psychiatry,* 1997. 38(4): p. 413-20.

[36] Chambers, W.J., et al., Psychotic symptoms in prepubertal major depressive disorder. *Arch Gen Psychiatry,* 1982. 39(8): p. 921-7.

[37] Famularo, R., R. Kinscherff, and T. Fenton, Psychiatric diagnoses of maltreated children: preliminary findings. *J Am Acad Child Adolesc Psychiatry,* 1992. 31(5): p. 863-7.

[38] Mundy, P., et al., The prevalence of psychotic symptoms in homeless adolescents. *J Am Acad Child Adolesc Psychiatry,* 1990. 29(5): p. 724-31.

[39] Sham, P.C., et al., Schizophrenia: sex and familial morbidity. *Psychiatry Res,* 1994. 52(2): p. 125-34.

[40] II, G., *Schizophrenia Genesis: The Origins of Madness.* 1991, New York: Freeman.

[41] van Os, J., et al., Prevalence of psychotic disorder and community level of psychotic symptoms: an urban-rural comparison. *Arch Gen Psychiatry,* 2001. 58(7): p. 663-8.

[42] Ryan, N.D., et al., The clinical picture of major depression in children and adolescents. *Arch Gen Psychiatry,* 1987. 44(10): p. 854-61.

[43] Kotsopoulos, S., et al., Hallucinatory experiences in nonpsychotic children. *J Am Acad Child Adolesc Psychiatry,* 1987. 26(3): p. 375-80.

[44] Apter, A., A. Bleich, and S. Tyano, Affective and psychotic psychopathology in hospitalized adolescents. *J Am Acad Child Adolesc Psychiatry,* 1988. 27(1): p. 116-20.

[45] Schreier, H.A., Auditory hallucinations in nonpsychotic children with affective syndromes and migraines: report of 13 cases. *J Child Neurol,* 1998. 13(8): p. 377-82.

[46] Ulloa, R.E., et al., Psychosis in a pediatric mood and anxiety disorders clinic: phenomenology and correlates. *J Am Acad Child Adolesc Psychiatry,* 2000. 39(3): p. 337-45.

[47] Mertin P, H.S., Auditory Hallucinations in Nonpsychotic Children: Diagnostic Considerations. *Child and Adolescent Mental Health,* 2004. 9(1): p. 9-14.

[48] Askenazy, F.L., et al., Auditory hallucinations in pre-pubertal children. A one-year follow-up, preliminary findings. *Eur Child Adolesc Psychiatry,* 2007. 16(6): p. 411-5.

[49] Best, N.T. and P. Mertin, Correlates of auditory hallucinations in nonpsychotic children. *Clin Child Psychol Psychiatry,* 2007. 12(4): p. 611-23.

[50] W, H. (2006) The mental health risks of adolescent cannabis use. *PLoS Med.* Volume,

[51] Putnam, F.W., Dissociative disorders in children: behavioral profiles and problems. *Child Abuse Negl,* 1993. 17(1): p. 39-45.

[52] Livingston, R., L. Lawson, and J.G. Jones, Predictors of self-reported psychopathology in children abused repeatedly by a parent. *J Am Acad Child Adolesc Psychiatry,* 1993. 32(5): p. 948-53.

[53] Ellason, J.W. and C.A. Ross, Childhood trauma and psychiatric symptoms. *Psychol Rep,* 1997. 80(2): p. 447-50.

[54] Kelleher I, H.M., Lynch F, Arseneault L, Fitzpatrick C, Cannon M, Associations between childhood trauma, bullying and psychotic symptoms among a school-based adolescent sample. *British Journal of Psychiatry,* In press.

[55] Janssen, I., et al., Childhood abuse as a risk factor for psychotic experiences. *Acta Psychiatr Scand,* 2004. 109(1): p. 38-45.

[56] Read, J., et al., Childhood trauma, psychosis and schizophrenia: a literature review with theoretical and clinical implications. *Acta Psychiatr Scand,* 2005. 112(5): p. 330-50.

[57] Burke, P., et al., Hallucinations in children. *J Am Acad Child Psychiatry,* 1985. 24(1): p. 71-5.

[58] Arseneault, L., et al., Bullying victimization uniquely contributes to adjustment problems in young children: a nationally representative cohort study. *Pediatrics,* 2006. 118(1): p. 130-8.

[59] Bowers L, S.P., Binney V, Perceived family relationships of bullies, victims and bully/victims in middle childhood. *Journal of Social and Personal Relationships,* 1994. 11(2): p. 215-232.

[60] Wessely, S., et al., Schizophrenia and Afro-Caribbeans. A case-control study. *Br J Psychiatry,* 1991. 159: p. 795-801.

[61] Van, O.J., et al., Psychotic illness in ethnic minorities: clarification from the 1991 census. *Psychol Med,* 1996. 26(1): p. 203-8.

[62] Tolmac, J. and M. Hodes, Ethnic variation among adolescent psychiatric in-patients with psychotic disorders. *Br J Psychiatry,* 2004. 184: p. 428-31.

[63] Laurens, K.R., et al., Psychotic-like experiences and other antecedents of schizophrenia in children aged 9-12 years: a comparison of ethnic and migrant groups in the United Kingdom. *Psychol Med,* 2007: p. 1-9.

[64] Patino, L.R., et al., Migration, family dysfunction and psychotic symptoms in children and adolescents. *Br J Psychiatry,* 2005. 186: p. 442-3.

[65] Escher, S., et al., Independent course of childhood auditory hallucinations: a sequential 3-year follow-up study. *Br J Psychiatry Suppl,* 2002. 43: p. s10-8.

[66] Hanssen, M., et al., The incidence and outcome of subclinical psychotic experiences in the general population. *Br J Clin Psychol,* 2005. 44(Pt 2): p. 181-91.

[67] Correll, C.U., et al., Prospective study of adolescents with subsyndromal psychosis: characteristics and outcome. *J Child Adolesc Psychopharmacol,* 2005. 15(3): p. 418-33.

[68] Garralda, M.E., Hallucinations in children with conduct and emotional disorders: II. The follow-up study. *Psychol Med,* 1984. 14(3): p. 597-604.

[69] Achenbach, *Manual for the Youth Self-Report and 1991 profile.* 1991, Burlington, VT: University of Vermont, Department of Psychiatry.

[70] Robins, L.N., et al., The Composite International Diagnostic Interview. An epidemiologic Instrument suitable for use in conjunction with different diagnostic systems and in different cultures. *Arch Gen Psychiatry,* 1988. 45(12): p. 1069-77.

[71] Schreier, H.A., Hallucinations in nonpsychotic children: more common than we think? *J Am Acad Child Adolesc Psychiatry,* 1999. 38(5): p. 623-5.

[72] Hermesh, H., et al., Musical hallucinations: prevalence in psychotic and nonpsychotic outpatients. *J Clin Psychiatry,* 2004. 65(2): p. 191-7.

[73] Cougnard, A., et al., Does normal developmental expression of psychosis combine with environmental risk to cause persistence of psychosis? A psychosis proneness-persistence model. *Psychol Med,* 2007. 37(4): p. 513-27.

[74] Bijl, R.V., A. Ravelli, and G. van Zessen, Prevalence of psychiatric disorder in the general population: results of The Netherlands Mental Health Survey and Incidence Study (NEMESIS). *Soc Psychiatry Psychiatr Epidemiol,* 1998. 33(12): p. 587-95.

[75] Bijl, R.V., et al., The Netherlands Mental Health Survey and Incidence Study (NEMESIS): objectives and design. *Soc Psychiatry Psychiatr Epidemiol,* 1998. 33(12): p. 581-6.

[76] Lieb, R., et al., The Early Developmental Stages of Psychopathology Study (EDSP): a methodological update. *Eur Addict Res,* 2000. 6(4): p. 170-82.

[77] Houston, J.E., et al., Childhood sexual abuse, early cannabis use, and psychosis: testing an interaction model based on the National Comorbidity Survey. *Schizophr Bull,* 2008. 34(3): p. 580-5.

[78] Bebbington PE, N.T., The Psychosis Screening Questionnaire. *International Journal of Methods in Psychiatric Research,* 1995. 5: p. 11-19.

[79] Shaffer, D., et al., The NIMH Diagnostic Interview Schedule for Children Version 2.3 (DISC-2.3): description, acceptability, prevalence rates, and performance in the MECA Study. Methods for the Epidemiology of Child and Adolescent Mental Disorders Study. *J Am Acad Child Adolesc Psychiatry,* 1996. 35(7): p. 865-77.

[80] Miller TJ, C.D., Markovich PJ et al, The SIPS screen: a brief self-report to detect the schizophrenia prodrome. *Schiophr Res*, 2004. 70(Suppl.): p. 78.

[81] Morrison, A.P., et al., Cognitive therapy for the prevention of psychosis in people at ultra-high risk: randomised controlled trial. *Br J Psychiatry,* 2004. 185: p. 291-7.

[82] Renton J, M.A., Effectiveness of cognitive therapy for psychosis and implications for early intervention. *Schizophrenia Research,* 2004. 70(1): p. 1-42.

[83] Morrison, A.P., et al., Three-year follow-up of a randomized controlled trial of cognitive therapy for the prevention of psychosis in people at ultrahigh risk. *Schizophr Bull,* 2007. 33(3): p. 682-7.

[84] McGlashan, T.H., et al., Randomized, double-blind trial of olanzapine versus placebo in patients prodromally symptomatic for psychosis. *Am J Psychiatry,* 2006. 163(5): p. 790-9.

[85] McGlashan, T.H., et al., The PRIME North America randomized double-blind clinical trial of olanzapine versus placebo in patients at risk of being prodromally symptomatic for psychosis. I. Study rationale and design. *Schizophr Res,* 2003. 61(1): p. 7-18.

[86] McGorry, P.D., et al., Randomized controlled trial of interventions designed to reduce the risk of progression to first-episode psychosis in a clinical sample with subthreshold symptoms. *Arch Gen Psychiatry,* 2002. 59(10): p. 921-8.

[87] McGorry PD, Y.A., Phillips LJ, Yuen HP, Francey S, Cosgrave EM, Germano D, Bravin J, McDonald T, Blair A, Adlard S, Jackson H, Marshall M, Rathbone J (2006) *Early Intervention for psychosis.* Volume, Issue 4, Art. No: CD004718 DOI: 10.1002/14651858

[88] Krabbendam, L., et al., Explaining transitions over the hypothesized psychosis continuum. *Aust N Z J Psychiatry,* 2005. 39(3): p. 180-6.

In: Adolescent Schizophrenia
Editors: J. T. Nillinghouse and R. P. Trotman

ISBN: 978-1-60692-370-2

Chapter IV

Psychoanalytical Teamwork on Schizophrenic Young Patients in a Day-hospital (Revisiting Some Developmental Pre-conditions for Patient's Subjective Appropriation)

Bernard Penot
Paris Psychoanalytical Institute, Paris, France

Abstract

Psychoanalytical psychotherapeutic "teamwork" may be recommended for dealing with this particular kind of mental pathology characterized by schizophrenic symptoms in young patients. In such cases, the degree of alienation is such that repetition is usually induced in other people (the therapists), filling in for fantasy construction that seems then to be lacking in the patient's psyche. A case like that of "Angel" can give some idea of this phenomenon, wherein several caregivers have to harbor fragmented and incompatible elements of the case's particular history, which are in need of more mental representation. Any subjective restitution and appropriation of these elements by the patient would require a sort of detour (often a trying one!) by way of the psychical space of caregivers whose initial task will be to "work it through" among themselves.

Keywords: Construction, restitution, passivation, subjectivation, disavowal, foreclosure, fantasy, transference, schizophenia, team work, clinical synthesis

The following considerations are based on my thirty years' practice as a psychiatrist in a day hospital, working with very disturbed adolescents who are not intellectually deficient.

What I want to illustrate here is one way that a psychoanalyst can be involved in an institutional setting, which consists of helping different team members to gain a better understanding of the *transference relation* they may be caught up in, whatever their professional role in the daily therapeutic program.

Lacan (1968) was certainly right to characterize the psychoanalyst's most specific action as "supporting the transference", and to consider it a way of allowing the patient to appropriate subjectively the conditions of his/her existence. But first I must specify *what kind of transference* we're dealing with here, and explain why it could be advisable to analyze it together as a team.

Adolescents who are admitted to a day-hospital for long-term treatment present pathological states essentially characterized, on the one hand, by disorders of the thought processes, with logical disturbances that can run to various forms of *hallucinatory delusion*; and on the other hand, by *conduct disorders* (a kind of delusion in the form of action) associated with many "borderline" pathologies. To the psychoanalyst, such symptoms appear to keep the patient in a state of subjective dispossession different from the kind produced by *repression* in neurotics, for they point to a *defect in the process of symbolization* that stands in the way of subjective recognition and appropriation.

The mechanism at work here is in fact *rejection from the thinkable* (Freud, 1918), which deprives perceptive representations of their possible signification, but without erasing them, as would occur with repression. The main effect of such rejection from signification is to defuse any affective charge the representation could give rise to, at most reducing it to the *uncanny* (Freud, 1919). But such rejection from symbolic play also tends to cause the disappearance of the very *subject* of any possible qualitative or attributive judgment. "No judgment is made, properly speaking", says Freud of such rejection-disavowal in the case of the Wolf Man.

The problem with our young day-hospital patients is that the psychoanalyst may wait in vain for their speech in session to provide the keys to understanding the troubles they are so visibly suffering. For they seem to have been deprived of the very roots needed to produce such speech. In fact, if we try as psychoanalysts to treat delusive or behavioral pathologies merely by means of a strict listening technique, taking into consideration only what the patient can verbalize in sessions, we risk looking like the fellow in an old joke, stubbornly looking for his lost keys in the area lit by a lamppost – not because he has any reason to think he lost them there, but just because that's where the light is !…

With patients whose psychical economy appears to be dominated by *rejection* and *disavowal-splitting*, a transference usually occurs that is not determined by fantasies. Insofar as fantasy representation has not been constructed in that point, the transference tends to take on an aspect of pure *acted repetition*: a stark re-actualization, within the therapeutic relation, of raw perceptive experiences "printed" as such in the patient's mind without having acquired the status of fantasy representation. I think we should certainly not consider fantasy organization as a given, automatically present at the outset of any mental life.

In my long-term work with such seriously alienated adolescents, I could regularly observe that the points where their thinking appeared to stop corresponded with areas that had been problematic for their family, particularly their parents. One will detect certain thought-blockages in the latter: they have trouble producing a discourse recounting some trials in their own history. This is due to a kind of narcissistic defense that forms a protective barrier against a traumatic experience, a wound which is felt at some generational level within the family. Indeed, the members of any "parental" generation (familial, national, etc.) can only put their own history into speech if they are willing to take a critical approach, to recognize the *lacks* and *shortcomings* which must have punctuated their history. But this sort of faultfinding cannot help but provoke certain narcissistic defenses aimed at sealing off traumatic experiences that could wound imaginary self-esteem.

This kind of defensive rejection within a multi-generational group mainly takes the form of a *community of disavowal (of signification),* which tends to deprive the latest generation of some speech connections necessary for situating and taking charge of its own existential genesis (Penot, 1998). We could say of such a family that it has failed to make enough myths (in ancient Greek, the word *muthos* merely means speech, discourse), in that it has not fostered the bonds of meaning that are indispensable for a subjective appropriation of the elements of its historical heritage.

This generational view of our young patients' troubles points to the idea of an *original active matrix of significations* which every new human being must have at the outset in order to compose an interior discourse and a fantasy life for himself. (what Lacan pleasantly called a "*ready-to-fantasize*"). All evidence suggests that this primary matrix is formed at the start of each individual life in the interactions between mother and baby – within what D. W. Winnicott (1975) proposed to call a *transitional space.* The mother's verbal and gestural responses to the earliest manifestations of the newborn organism's drives will provide elements of signification that will gradually become recognizable for the latter.

Whence Lacan's key idea that the *signifiers* the subject can refer to emanate first from the primal (parental) Other (Lacan, 1964).

I have been struck by the fact the only text where Freud is willing to employ the term *subject* in a systematic way is none other than "Instincts [drives] and their Vicissitudes" (1915).[1] As far as I know, this fact has not been touched upon ; nor has it been noted that Freud uses first the term *subject* here to designate an *exterior suject*: a drive agent capable of satisfying the baby's need to be looked at and to be handled. (Curiously, Freud omits the need to be listened to.) The formula "to get something done (to oneself)" that Freud uses here best renders the always active character of the drive, even when it is seeking to be satisfied in a passive way. André Green (1980) proposed that this active seeking be called "*passivation*"; different from passivity, it could connote the "feminine" drive activity in both sexes.[2]

These considerations led me to propose (Penot, 2001) a psychoanalytical definition of the subject as a *drive agent caught up in a signifying relation.* This conception of a drive subject

[1] Strachey is obviously attached to a systematic use of the terms *subject* and *object* within a univocal polarity in which the *subject* is always supposed to correspond to the own-person. It is thus striking to see how, in "Instincts [drives] and their vicissitudes" (1915), he doesn't strictly follow Freud's use of the term *Subjekt* ; he confusingly uses the English word *subject* three times when Freud doesn't, speaking of: "*the subject's own self*", (p. 126, 127) and "*subject's own body*" (p. 129) This makes it difficult to follow in English Freud's revolutionary idea of a necessary "time" during which an external drive agent, thus designated as *subject*, must be "put in place", outside, by the own-person to satisfy his drive aim of being treated as an object.

[2] Green says (p. 186): "*L'action de la pulsion, elle-même active, 'passivise' le sujet qui la subit* " – [the action of the drive, which is in itself active, 'passivates' the subject that undergoes it (my translation).]

captures very well the exemplary character of the subjective threshold of adolescence – if we consider the latter as a change in the drive regimen, requiring a calling into question of the signifying subjective references established during childhood.

Anyway, it seems to me that one advantage of this model of the primary role of a signifying Other is that it points to the kind of therapeutic setting best-suited to dealing with severe problems of subjectivation. This term has been proposed by André Green (1980). I consider that it designates the most specific aim of any psychoanalytic work (individual or not), whose *aim-representation* is the subjective appropriation by the patient of the elements of his/her life. This is what differentiates the psychoanalytical method from behavioral and cognitivist ones, starting with Freud's first remarks to Dora.

In a classical treatment setting, an analyst must not be afraid to take on the demanding role of the patient's primal Other – as I have suggested in my account of the treatment of a bulimic (Penot, 2001). But young patients in a day hospital oblige us to go back even further in the genesis of the process of subjectivation – to a stage Melanie Klein, with remarkable intuition, designated as the *paranoid schizoid position,* the therapeutic *reprise* of which can at first take place only through a "transference" that is fragmentary, diffracted onto several protagonists.

Thus, a therapeutic institution that purports to help youngsters surmount serious subjective troubles must first of all comprise not only a place for speaking, in sessions and technical acts (as frequent as these may be) but also *a space for living together and enabling exchangeable speech to be born out of experiences lived together* – in short, a space that allows for mythmaking (discourse making)... But if the team of care-givers are to foster nascent speech in this way, they should not limit themselves to sharing activities of daily life with the youngsters. They must also be ready to serve as supports for the *transference reproduction,* within the institutional milieu, of certain defects inherent to each case, and to recognize these re-actualizations in their daily contact with the patient.

Psychoanalytical Teamwork

As soon as an adolescent with a psychical breakdown has been admitted to the day hospital, his investment of (and by) the therapeutic milieu will generally be signaled by a very characteristic phenomenon. During our weekly work in the team meeting called the *clinical synthesis,* we will be able to detect a startling clash of viewpoints among the caregivers in charge (we call them *referents*) of the case in question. Colleagues who usually get along well together suddenly start suspecting each other of incompetence or worse…

This is usually perceived not so much in the conflict between subjective positions, but rather in their *incompatibility*, and in the surprising inability of each person involved to identify with another's point of view, even though they have worked closely together for a long time. We are then obliged to work with this kind of subjective positioning, which places us in a mutual relationship of *rejection-exclusion* and *disqualification*. The virulence of this phenomenon of reciprocal invalidation usually turns out to be in proportion to the degree of psychosis of the case.

Since the early seventies, our regular observation of this phenomenon has led us, as a team, to adopt the methodology of dealing with it as a particular kind of *transference* – in other words, as a displacement *(Übertragung)* into our therapeutic community of existential relationships that may have presided over the primary genesis of the case in its original matrix.

This idea can at least help us to stand the phenomenon, which is always very trying at first. Indeed, it is essential that we refrain as much as possible from trying to resolve these difficulties by determining who is "right" and who is "wrong" – in other words, it is important to suspend the *attributive-condemning judgment* that Freud (Negation, 1925) specifically designates as the mechanism by which the Ego is circumscribed.

For this kind of work, it is indispensable that each team member, whatever his function, be able to express freely, without fear of attributive *ad hominem* judgment, the unexpected subjective role that he finds himself having to play. When our team *synthesis* manages to function from this perspective (and the head doctor must ensure this), various experiences, even shocking ones, can be expressed without too much trouble, or at least without hampering our collaborative work of thought and research.

If the team is to function in this way, its hierarchy (of physicians, psychoanalysts...) must be suspended, as much as possible, at least during the time of clinical synthesis.[3] It may seem paradoxical that psychoanalytical work (analyzing transference and working it through) could involve all the caregivers on the team – a majority of whom are non-analysts, and many of whom are not even analyzed... There has, of course, to be a consensus about this among the team members.

We must also be in agreement about another basic idea: that we can only work through what has been sufficiently re-actualized in the treatment setting and lived through by the caregivers. So we think it would be counterproductive to try to avoid any "traumatic repetition" with the young patient (rather like trying to avoid transference in a standard psychoanalysis!) On the contrary, we consider that the odd subjective attitudes manifested by different caregivers provide precious clues about what is at issue with the patient.

Using the Term "Projection"

Here I should explain why I prefer to avoid using the term "projection", or "projective identification" to describe the kind of transference we are dealing with as a team. It is because I think that words in themselves carry implicit representations, even, I would say, an implicit philosophy. The term *projection* cannot help but suggest an *imaginary* process – while it is my conviction that the phenomenon I am talking about is mainly the result of a *lack* of mental imagery, more precisely of organized fantasy in the patient's psyche.

The mechanism of projective identification was introduced by Melanie Klein in 1946. However, she envisioned it as the projection of a fantasy intolerable for the patient's ego into

[3] This is the reason why I prefer to use the term "team" here, rather than "staff", which implies a hierachical structure.

the psyche of the therapist. Fortunately, many "post-Kleinian" authors have considerably transformed the content of the notion of projective identification.

Bion went furthest in re-defining it. I think that, while he uses other terms, his theoretical line most converges with the one I am proposing here on the basis of other sources. When, for example, Bion speaks of "undigested parts of [the patient's] experience" (1967), he is obviously speaking of what I call perceptual traces (prints) lacking mental representation. And he helped projective identification to be viewed, not only as a defense in the service of (ego) mis-recognition, but also as a way of experiencing something in need of more mental representation.

The Interaction with the Family

If we compare the subjective material from our team synthesis with what we know about the patient's family, it helps to diffuse somewhat the virulence of inter-personal tensions within the team – enabling each of us to live with these divergent (incompatible) experiences and let them be played out, to *host* them long enough for them to be articulated into conflict that can be verbalized. The concomitant work of the caregivers with each family usually helps us to link our surprising experiences with attitudes particular to the family itself.[4]

The important thing is that what is thus transferred into our midst is in sum a *rejection-disavowal (Verleugnung)* that probably played a decisive role in the first entourage of the young person in question. This occurs through what I proposed to call the *automatism of repetition induced in the other.* Unlike object transference, this phenomenon is not determined by the patient's fantasy organization, even unconscious. On the contrary, we usually observe that such induction in the other will be all the more inevitable insofar as it corresponds to a *lack* of fantasy construction in the patient, at least in a certain sector of his psyche.

It is my hypothesis that this phenomenon of induction leads to an actualization, within the therapeutic relation, of *early perceptive imprints* that could not acquire enough mental imagery. Does this perhaps give an idea of the psychical register Lacan called "*le Réel*"?[5] The fact remains that the psychical work must first be done *among therapists*.[6] Their work of putting these early perceptive experience into representations and into words tends to result

[4] We have opted for a system wherein family therapies are conducted by the psychiatrist and the male-female couple of "referents" (psychologist/educator) who are in charge of the patient on a daily basis.

[5] The two other registers Lacan conceptualized are "l'Imaginaire", which corresponds more or less to Freud's *thing representations*, and "le Symbolique", which is made up of "signifiers" and *word representations.* Lacan's "Réel" consists of unsymbolized perceptions; it is a register of the psyche and must not be confused with the reality that biologists or physicists deal with: it is made up of perceptive memory without psychical imagery.

[6] We also observe, of course, some kinds of transferential effects onto other patients, but these cannot be analyzed, elaborated and used in the same way as transference onto caregivers..

in a certain "*restitution*"[7] for the youngster of the missing signifying references he needs to structure his singular experience.

It is as though such a detour through the other/caregiver, along with the latter's methodical work of auto-acknowledgement, makes possible a putting into images and words that had been unattainable for the patient, and enables him to subjectively appropriate new tools of mental representation for his own use. It is logical to refrain from addressing any interpretation directly to the patient at this stage, which we could consider *pre-subjective*. But we will often observe a noticeable improvement in his psychotic or behavioral symptoms at this time, as if the strict repetition determinism had already been overcome by the mere fact of being recognized and borne by the caregivers for the necessary time, before perhaps being put back into the *circuit* (of speech) in family therapy.

I think that the psychoanalytical term "*counter-transference*" does not adequately describe this phenomenon of induction in the other/caregiver. For it was coined by Freud to connote the psychoanalyst's subjective reaction to a *fantasy projection* made onto him by the patient, who treats the analyst as an "object" of his/her unconscious fantasy. The phenomenon we are describing here belongs to a very different register where fantasy has not been constituted.

It is then through the short-circuiting of his own *pre-conscious* system that the therapist will first find himself caught up in the *repetition determinism* when in contact with the case. Once we are able to learn something of certain psychotics' prior institutional treatments, we cannot help but be struck by the series of remarkably similar reactions induced in those (even very different) people who have treated them. This is like the oft-observed experience of some abused children who have been removed from their parents and placed in foster care: the foster parents may also begin to beat the child, even if they have never before harmed any of their charges… Dr Xavier Jacquey was the first to suggest (in agreement with François Perrier) that such a subjective position induced in the therapist be called "*subjectal transference*"[8]. I would argue that, within this kind of transference, the therapist is positioned as primal exterior drive agent (Freud, 1915) "commanding" the nascent subject.

This is a good reason, I think, for adopting a setting that would allow several caregivers to analyze together the effects of this transference. Collaboration acts as a check on each person's spontaneous tendency to feel a priori that his/her own reaction to the case is adequate ("professional"). In some exceptional cases, an analyst working alone with a psychotic patient may perceive how he/she has been caught up in subjective repetition (as happened with some pioneering psychoanalysts). But this is usually easier to perceive when one is working with other therapists; for it is the observation of the caregivers' very different subjective positions that underscore for all of them how partial and debatable their initial attitudes can be.

---

[7] For this, Freud chose the term *Wiederhersztellung* on the last page of "Constructions in the Analysis" (1937); but Strachey missed its specific meaning when he merely translated it as "*cure*" ! (S. E. XXIII, p. 268)

[8] JACQUEY, X. 1972: "De l'analyse des phénomènes contre-transférentiels en termes de contre-attitudes dans le champ psychothérapique institutionnel ; contribution au traitement des psychotiques" [On the analysis of counter-transferential attitudes in terms of counter-attitudes in the institutional

The Model of Psychoanalytical Psychodrama and the Purloined Letter

What first led me to recognize the importance of this particular kind of transference, usually misunderstood in institutions, was my practice of *psychoanalytical psychodrama* in the seventies (with one patient, one leader and several therapists improvising the play). While leading a session of psychodrama with a psychotic adolescent, I was rather astonished to see how one or another of my fellow "players", who knew nearly nothing about the patient and his family, would spontaneously incorporate into his playacting attitudes that *I* knew to be characteristic of one of the patient's parents – even to the point of reproducing specific intonations! This "information" could only have been transmitted through the patient himself, though he was nearly mute. But how? We came to understand that this enigmatic (to say the least) phenomenon was occurring throughout our institutional work.

This view helps us to *detach* ourselves imaginarily, to put into perspective the virulence of team relationships necessarily perceived *a priori* as personal. It makes it easier for the professionals on the team to take on antagonistic roles as if they were their own, for as long as necessary, to become their *hosts,* long enough to be able to articulate them into conflict that can be put into dialectic and elaborated.

This leads me to clarify something about the *setting necessary for such work.* I have suggested considering the Lacan's famous commentary on Poe's "The Purloined Letter" as providing a representative model of what we are dealing with.[9] For the subjective positions of the protagonists, in the successive scenes of the story, appear to be determined by the relationship that each one maintains with the compromising object.

We can thus detect several series of "castings" involving the subjective roles surrounding this object (letter) which is both enigmatic and compromising (like the psychotic). But the determinism of the distribution of roles *"would remain invisible to the audience"*, Lacan emphasizes, without the narrative process set in motion by Poe. This seems to me analogous with the necessity for a certain kind of *clinical synthesis* to enable us, working as a team, to put into words the transference's "cast of characters", often observed in the case of psychotics, but just as often misunderstood.

Physicists know better than anyone (apparently better than many psychiatrists!) how the methodological set-up that we use determines what we will be able to observe.

These subjective positions are characteristically experienced *a priori* by those who occupy them as having an objective, professional basis. It is thanks to an arrangement enabling them to be confronted with each other that their strange incompatibility can be perceived for what it is: *a developed, projected formula of disavowal-splitting which is inherent to the case.*

I would add that similar phenomena of repetitive induction can of course be observed outside of dysfunctional families or teamwork in a day hospital. Our colleague Vamik Volkan (1997) has remarkably described collective behaviors throughout the world which may be

psychotherapeutic field ; a contribution to the treatment of psychotics], unpubished doctoral dissertation in medecine, Paris, Salpétrière

[9] Even if Lacan himself had other aims in mind when he proposed this commentary.

considered « delusive ». Indeed, in some ethnic communities (Bosnia, Africa, etc.), it is through the generational transmission of some traumatic historical references has been frozen, or fossilized, making these elements resistant to any symbolic elaboration or transformation – only able to induce a blind behavioral repetition (mostly a violent one).

In addition, it is interesting to note that each professional's degree of clear-sightedness depends not so much (at least at the beginning) on his/her competence or psychoanalytical training, but rather on the *transferential position* he/she holds in relation to the case: a position which determines the mode of subjective involvement, and the blind spots that go with it.[10] Such an observation could justify our working psychoanalytically with non-analysts – and I would add that resistance to this view tends to arise more on the part of (some) analysts...

The Case of "Angel"

I will try to illustrate this briefly with the case of an adolescent we received at the age of fourteen, arriving with a label of "entry into schizophrenia" and a prescription for Haldol. He had been adopted at the end of his first year by a bourgeois Parisian couple, when it appeared that the husband's low sperm count would prevent them from ever having a baby.

Something in the circumstances of this boy's breakdown struck me right away: it had followed the unexpected discovery of jaundice due to a benign congenital liver condition. The teenager had then begun to manifest intense anxiety with psychotic overtones, becoming extremely aggressive and rejecting towards his adoptive parents. He was expelled from his school, then refused by another, before coming to our institution where he would be treated for three years.

I wondered about the strangely destabilizing power of this congenital stigma: a sudden re-apparition of his biological parents (real, yet unknown), a signifier of something of the boy's biological origin. His adoptive mother kept insisting: "For me, it's exactly as if I had given birth to him"... Striving to reconstitute her son's early childhood for me, irreproachable medical records in hand, she said that though a very beautiful baby, he was "perhaps a little stiff, tense". Then the father chimes in with, "he was suspicious!"

This remarkable parental reaction (here, I would be tempted to speak of a projection *onto the son) hints at an adoptive parent's own suspicious gaze upon this seed sprung from who-knows-where (a suspicion that had found confirmation in the appearance of the congenital stigma?) The father later gave evidence of quite remarkable projective attitudes regarding the rightwing extremist views expressed by the son: "He has pretty radical ideas about his fellow human beings. If it were up to him, there'd be fewer people on Earth!" said this infertile man.*

Once he was admitted to our day hospital, this handsome boy would show himself to be more perverse than schizophrenic. I will call him "Angel", after the ambiguous, seductive

[10] This characteristic led me to refer to the Lacan's commentary on Poe's "The Purloined Letter" as best able to shed light on this kind of fundamentally unconscious phenomenon (Lacan J. *Ecrits*, édit. Du Seuil, Paris, 1966, p.7)

angel in Pasolini's film "Theoreme". We had first of all to overcome the destructive effects of incompatible feelings that arose among the caregivers after coming into contact with this strange boy. Everyone's experiences tended to be mutually exclusive, along the lines of a disavowal, within a team that had been working rather well together for a long time.

Only during Angel's second year of hospitalization did his psychologist-referent begin to overcome her "embarrassment" enough to be able to verbalize in our clinical synthesis the uneasiness she was prey to when she found herself alone in a room with Angel. She said that she would then feel in danger of fainting, of blacking out, that her thinking was completely baffled. It is noteworthy that at such times she never even thought of calling out to a colleague within earshot. This reminds me of what Freud says about the childhood experience of the "Wolf Man"(1918), who was hallucinating that his finger had been severed and yet could not call out to his Nanny, who was close by.

So there seemed to be something unnamable, impossible to formulate, that had to be lived through. The violence of such an experience was all the more striking in that it involved a seasoned psychologist, who was also a former nurse. In addition, there was a striking contrast with the attitudes of other female team members towards Angel: another psychologist willingly let him nuzzle up against her neck, certain that this was simply the innocent manifestation of a little boy who, she said, "didn't get enough cuddling". But others did not like having to witness such scenes, which they found "perverse".

The male team members were also divided into violently clashing subjective positions. Angel's educator-referent complained of feeling constantly disavowed – "couillonné" *was the word he kept using (a mildly vulgar expression meaning "to be made a fool of", but whose literal connotations refer to the testicles, or "balls"). Another male colleague, however, used to speak of his "positive relationship" with this boy, who moved him to solicitude.*

Our psychoanalytical teamwork, as we confronted these "impossible" relationships created between caregivers, was aimed at putting them (laboriously) into words for ourselves – in the form of hypotheses, in the sense of what Freud calls "Constructions in the analysis" (1937). We know how sometimes a virulent imaginary disqualification of the biological parents can prevail in the minds of troubled adoptive parents. This state of mind (especially when it is unconscious) tends to have a destructive effect on the adopted child. His narcissistic references may boomerang between the "nasty abandoners" and the "child-stealers". Adoptive parents may have even more reason to blacken the hypothetical image of the biological parents (the "real" parents, as they are bizarrely called) when they are having trouble exercising their own parental function.

One day in the synthesis, Angel's psychologist-referent finally expressed, not without anger and resentment, that in her work with Angel, she felt like "a woman without enough protection." (sic). She was then able to realize the extent to which she had found herself locked into the probable experience of the ghostly, unknown biological mother – as if she were the Dibbuk[11] *of a real being that has been abolished, leaving no words or image – in other words, foreclosed.*

As a result of this process of mentalization going on around him, Angel gradually managed to improve his behavior, and to develop a fantasy life, inventing a family romance

[11] This form of ghostly return of a misunderstood dead person is well-known in kabbalistic tradition.

about an Anglo-Saxon origin (made plausible by his ginger hair and freckles.) He insisted on adopting an English nickname, "Bad luck". Which makes one wonder: bad luck for whom? For himself, because of the way he'd turned out? For his biological parents, because they could not assume responsibility for his birth? For his adoptive parents, because they were dealt such a bad hand? For us, finally, because we had to deal with this difficult case?...

Then Angel ran away from home to London, where he managed to live on his own for one week (establishing contact with his father by telephone). He came back expressing his satisfaction at having accomplished something personal, and was able to return more successfully to his secondary studies.

Only at the end of the treatment, could his mother reveal during a family session, and thus in Angel's presence, of course, that he had physically battered her after his breakdown. She had never breathed a word of this to her husband.

I happened to see this young man again, several years later. He came to ask me some questions about fatherhood, for at twenty-five, he already had a large family to take care of – having already managed to acquire two children and two stepchildren...

Perspectives

I have tried to illustrate a kind of psychoanalytical teamwork that I think most adequate for overcoming serious subjective disorders. It usually has to deal with a particular kind of *transference*, which I have called *repetition induced in the other.* In these cases dominated by a *foreclosure* of meaning, it proves necessary for the therapists to accept being caught up in that always surprising *repetition* through which such patients' early traumatic conditions tend to be re-actualized. It is by working through this particular *transference* that we can enable the patient to appropriate subjectively something in his life that *has already happened, but was not really experienced* (as Winnicott first formulated it), something that was inadequately symbolized and will therefore keep *coming back* in the form of hallucination or pathological behavior.

This relates to Freud's interest in *ghosts*. And it is indeed remarkable that, in popular tradition as well, ghostly re-apparitions have always been understood to be the consequence of a stifled truth, a disavowal of judgment which keeps demanding restitution.

Once the team confrontation has allowed each therapist to realize better how he/she has been caught against his will in the *repetition induced in the other,* it is possible to perceive how this kind of subjective hold differs structurally from the usual pre-conscious reactions of an analyst to the projected fantasies of patients on the couch.

But I think we should consider that such teamwork fundamentally belongs to a psychoanalytical perspective, insofar as the most specific aim of psychoanalytical activity is to foster the process of subjective appropriation. This is what Freud memorably summarized in his famous sentence: "*Wo es war, soll ich werden*" – literally, where *that* was, *I* should become.

And depending on the progress that a young patient may have made, through institutional treatment, towards a better subjective appropriation of "that" (Id) which had already happened in his life without being mentalized, it may be possible to advise him/her to undertake an individual treatment with a psychoanalyst.[12]

References

Bion, W. R. (1967) *Second Thoughts. Selected Papers on Psychoanalysis.* London, Heinemann.

Freud, S. 1915, "Instincts and their Vicissitudes", S.E. XIV, p. 111.

Freud, S. 1918, "From the History of an Infantile Neurosis", S.E. XVII, p. 3.

Freud, S. 1919, "The Uncanny", S. E. XVII, p. 219.

Freud, S. 1925, Negation, S.E. XIX, p. 235.

Green, A. 1980, "Passions et destins des passions" – *La folie privée,* Gallimard, 1990, p.186.

Kernberg, O. (1988) Projection and projective identification: developmental and clinical aspects. In *Projection, Identification, Projective Identification.* Ed. J. Sandler, Karnak, p. 93.

Klein, M. (1946) *Envy and Gratitude and Other Works.* Hogarth Press, 1975, p.141-175.

Lacan, J. 1954-55, Séminaire sur les Psychoses, édit. du Seuil, Paris.

Lacan, J. *Ecrits*, édit. Du Seuil, Paris, 1966, p.7

Penot, B. 1998, "Disavowal of reality as an act of filial piety", *Int. Journ.* Vol. 79, 1, p. 27.

Penot, B. 2001, "The drive circuit as generator of subjectivation", *Internat. Journ. of Psycho-Anal*, Vol. 82, n° 3, p. 501.

Rosenfeld, D. (1978) Notes on the psychopathology and psychoanalytic treatment of some borderline patients, *Int. J. Psychoanal. 59,* p. 215-221.

Volkan V. 1997, *Blood lines - from ethnic pride to ethnic terrorism*, Westview press USA.

Winnicott, D.W. (1963), "Dependence in infant care, in child care, and in the psycho-analytic setting", *Internat. Journ. of Psycho-Anal,* n°44, p.339-344. – (1971) *Playing and Reality*, London, Tavistock.

[12] Individual psychotherapy is usually prescribed at a second stage – except of course when the patient already had an outside psychotherapist at the time of admission. After one, two or three years of institutional treatment, individual sessions are frequently proposed with an analyst working in our day hospital.

In: Adolescent Schizophrenia
Editors: J. T. Nillinghouse and R. P. Trotman

ISBN: 978-1-60692-370-2

Chapter V

Treatment Approaches to Aggressive Behavior in Schizophrenia

Jan Volavka [*]
Nathan Kline Institute and New York University, NY, USA

Abstract

Treatment of psychiatric disorders is hampered by the fact that their causes are poorly understood. Our ignorance is even deeper when it comes to aggressive behavior in psychiatric patients. Clearly, without better understanding of underlying neuropsychobiology of aggression we cannot improve the existing treatments. This chapter therefore first reviews neurobiological and psychosocial factors affecting aggression in schizophrenia, and then proceeds to discuss their implications for treatment. Finally, the current state of the psychopharmacology of aggression in schizophrenia is briefly reviewed.

1. Neurobiological and Psychosocial Factors That Affect Aggression in Schizophrenia

Modern studies of the neurobiological factors that modulate aggressive and criminal behavior in humans rest largely on the innovative approaches pioneered by Sarnoff A. Mednick (Mednick and Volavka, 1980; Mednick, Pollock, Volavka, and Gabrielli, Jr., 1982; Mednick, Gabrielli, Jr., and Hutchings, 1983; Mednick, Gabrielli, Jr., and Hutchings, 1984; Mednick and Kandel, 1988). His contributions to our understanding of the neurobiology of schizophrenia, discussed elsewhere in this volume, are enormous. The study of the aggressive

[*] Email: janvolavka@gmail.com. Phone 406 995 2776. Mailing address: 55 Blue Spruce Road #E3, P.O. Box 160663, Big Sky, MT 59716-0663

behavior in schizophrenia, representing the confluence of these two lines of inquiry, has been heavily influenced by Mednick's thought, and many of the current outstanding researchers in the area had been his students.

Schizophrenia patients living in the community have an elevated risk for aggressive behavior in comparison with community residents who are not diagnosed with mental disorder (Swanson, Holzer, Ganju, and Jono, 1990). The elevated risk is present even if the patient has no comorbidity with other disorders (Swanson, 1994; Arseneault, Moffitt, Caspi, Taylor, and Silva, 2000; Brennan, Mednick, and Hodgins, 2000), and it is further elevated by comorbidities.

1.1. Comorbid Substance Use Disorders

The risk for aggressive behavior is increased, quite dramatically, with comorbid substance use disorders (Lindqvist and Allebeck, 1990; Swanson, 1994). Comorbidity of schizophrenia and substance use disorders is highly prevalent: almost 50% of schizophrenia patients have a comorbid substance use disorder, and schizophrenia patients are almost 5 times more likely to develop a substance use disorder than the rest of the population (the odds ratio was estimated at 4.6) (Regier et al., 1990). Therefore, the propensity of schizophrenia patients to abuse alcohol or drugs represents an important pathway towards the development of aggressive behavior. Furthermore, successful treatment of comorbid substance use disorders is expected to reduce aggressive behavior in schizophrenia patients.

1.2. Comorbid Personality Disorders

Personality disorders, particularly antisocial personality disorder (DSM-IV) or psychopathy (Hare, 1986) are associated with aggressive behavior in the general population (Volavka, 2002; Hart, Hare, and Forth, 1994). The relation between these two diagnoses is discussed elsewhere (Hare, 1996). Comorbidity of schizophrenia and personality disorders has not been studied with the same epidemiological rigor as the comorbidity with substance use disorders. However, limited data suggest that comorbidity of psychopathy and schizophrenia exists, and that it is higher among violent than among non-violent patients (Nolan, Volavka, Mohr, and Czobor, 1999). Comorbid psychopathy may thus be another risk factor for aggression in schizophrenia patients.

1.3. Treatment Non-Adherence

As we will see, antipsychotics possess varying degrees of antiaggressive effects in schizophrenia patients. It is therefore not surprising that the risk of aggressive behavior increases if the patient stops taking his medication. Thus, non-adherence to pharmacological treatment is another factor that elevates the risk of aggressive behavior (Swartz et al., 1998a;

Swartz et al., 1998b). Non-adherence to recommended antipsychotic treatment in the community occurs in a majority of patients (Dolder, Lacro, Dunn, and Jeste, 2002).

Non-adherence to antipsychotic medication regimens has many causes. Some of these are *drug-related*: the side effects may be difficult to tolerate. Such intolerable side effects may include extrapyramidal symptoms (more common with typical antipsychotics), weight gain (more common with atypicals, particularly clozapine and olanzapine) and sexual dysfunction related to prolactin elevation due to dopamine D2 receptor blocking (more common with typical antipsychotics and risperidone). Atypical antipsychotics appear to have a slightly better treatment adherence record than the typicals (Dolder et al., 2002), and clozapine has the best adherence overall. This may be due to the frequent mandatory blood tests; regular contacts with the treatment team maintain and strengthen treatment alliance; they also improve the monitoring of the patient. Slow-release injectable forms of antipsychotics are generally superior to the oral forms in terms of adherence (Swartz, Swanson, Wagner, Burns, and Hiday, 2001).

Other factors that may contribute to non-adherence involve *environmental influences, including treatment management.* The psychiatrist may not have established the appropriate treatment alliance with the patient, or may not have adequately explained the benefits of treatment and the risks of discontinuing it. The patient's family may not have been adequately informed about the treatment, or it chose not to be involved. Finally, non-adherence may be caused by *patient-related* factors. These include delusional beliefs about medication, inadequate insight or denial of mental illness, and cognitive problems that interfere with the patient's ability to understand and adhere to a treatment regimen. Non-adherence is frequently combined with comorbid substance abuse which may further impair patients' judgment and motivation.

1.4. Heterogeneity of Aggressive Behavior

Comorbid substance use disorders and non-adherence to treatment are important factors in the development of aggressive behavior in schizophrenia patients residing in the community. However, aggressive behavior occurs frequently even when substance use is precluded and treatment adherence is close to complete (Volavka, 2002). Such conditions can be created at psychiatric inpatient units. Overt physical aggression can be closely observed and studied prospectively at such units; the observations of individual aggressive incidents would not be feasible in the community.

It has long been assumed that aggression in psychiatric patients (and, more generally, in humans) is a heterogeneous phenomenon in terms of its causation and underlying neurobiology. Nevertheless, current research into the treatment of aggressive behavior tacitly assumes neurobiological and sociobiological homogeneity across all incidents of aggression: to assess treatment effect, the incidents are counted and their severity quantified, without any attempt at causative analysis. This shortcoming is understandable since empirical research addressing causative heterogeneity of aggressive incidents is sparse. Such research is important: if there are different causes, for example different neurobiological mechanisms, one would assume that the appropriate treatments might vary accordingly.

One of the ways to assess the heterogeneity of aggressive incidents is to observe them and to interview the participants and witnesses. We have installed a video camera system that is continuously recording the activity in the public areas of our research inpatient unit. The aggressive incidents that are captured are archived for further study. At a minimum, the video permits a reliable identification of the assailant and the victim. As soon as possible after the incident occurs, researchers interview the assailant, the victim, and any witnesses. A semi-structured interview was developed to assess the causal contributions of psychotic symptoms, disordered impulse control, and psychopathy to the observed aggressive incident. The data on 70 incidents were published (Nolan et al., 2003). The results indicated that approximately 20 percent of the assaults in this sample were directly related to positive psychotic symptoms. Factor analysis revealed two psychosis-related factors, one related to positive psychotic symptoms and the other to psychotic confusion and disorganization, as well as a third factor that differentiated impulsive from psychopathic assaults.

This information is potentially useful in the selection of rational antiaggressive treatment strategies: hypothetically, the psychosis-related assaults would respond to atypical antipsychotics, and impulse-control disorder assaults to adjunctive anticonvulsants. Psychopathy assaults might respond to an elaborate, long-term term cognitive-behavioral treatment that will be described below.

This study represents only a first step in the effort to understand the heterogeneity of aggressive behavior. We have collected additional data on aggressive incidents and replicated these results (Nolan et al., in preparation). However, we are still not sure that our classification of assaults will help to classify people. Such classification is of course important from the standpoint of treatment: we treat people, not assaults.

1.5. Genetics and Genomics

Genetics and genomics represent another approach to the analysis of aggressive behavior in schizophrenia that has potential therapeutic implications. Many neurotransmitter systems that are under partial genetic control play a role in the regulation of aggressive behavior; most research has focused on serotonin (Volavka, 2002). Recently, catecholamines such as dopamine and norepinephrine have been receiving increased attention. These substances enhance aggression in animals, and their antagonists (such as haloperidol and propranolol) are known to reduce certain types of aggressive behavior in humans (Volavka, 2002).

The major enzymes responsible for catecholamine catabolism are catechol-*O*-methyltransferase (COMT) and monoamine oxidase (MAO). A common biallelic single nucleotide polymorphism, involving a Met → Val substitution at codon 158 of the COMT gene has been identified at chromosome 22q11.1-q11.2 (Lachman et al., 1996). The methionine (Met) allele at this locus is associated with low enzymatic activity, whereas the valine (Val) allele is associated with high activity. Homozygosity for the Met allele yields a 3- to 4-fold reduction in COMT activity relative to Val homozygotes, with heterozygotes demonstrating intermediate activity.

If catecholamines enhance aggression and their antagonists suppress it, then the Met allele conferring low enzymatic activity of COMT should be associated with enhanced aggressive behavior because low catabolism of catecholamines leads to greater amounts of these compounds in the brain (and elsewhere). This prediction has been confirmed in some (Strous, Bark, Parsia, Volavka, and Lachman, 1997; Strous et al., 2003; Lachman, Nolan, Mohr, Saito, and Volavka, 1998; Kotler et al., 1999; Volavka et al., 2004b), but not all (Jones et al., 2001) studies of schizophrenia, schizoaffective disorder, and other disorders (Rujescu, Giegling, Gietl, Hartmann, and Moller, 2003).. Also consistent with the prediction, COMT knockout mice show elevated aggressive behavior (Gogos et al., 1998). Furthermore, when 8 inbred mouse strains were ranked by their aggressiveness, the ranking was inversely correlated with the expression of the COMT gene in the hippocampus: the lower the COMT expression, the higher the strain aggressiveness. (Fernandes et al., 2004).

Thus, the Met allele (and the attendant lowering of COMT activity) is associated with aggression. However, it is also associated with enhanced cognitive performance (Egan et al., 2001). This conjunction is counterintuitive, since elevated aggression is typically associated with low cognitive performance; higher intelligence is generally considered a protective factor against aggressive behavior (Volavka, 2002). Reconciling these findings is beyond the scope of this chapter; information can be found elsewhere (Bilder, Volavka, Lachman, and Grace, 2004).

2. Treatment Implications of the Neurobiological and Psychobiological Factors

2.1. Comorbid Substance Use Disorders

Schizophrenia patients with comorbid substance use disorders require services of integrated treatment teams that are equipped to approach both illnesses as primary targets of intervention. Since the comorbidity is so prevalent, the goal is to define all psychiatric programs as "dual diagnosis programs" and to make them capable to treat these difficult patients. Integrated philosophy of treatment is based on a disease and recovery model.

Continuing psychopharmacological treatment of schizophrenia is an integral part of the treatment.

There is some evidence suggesting that clozapine may reduce the drug and alcohol use in schizophrenia patients (Drake, Xie, McHugo, and Green, 2000). The mechanism of such effect is not clear. Perhaps clozapine treats a reward deficiency syndrome (Green, Zimmet, Strous, and Schildkraut, 1999), reduces craving (Buckley, McCarthy, Chapman, Richman, and Yamamoto, 2000), or its superior antipsychotic effect enables the patients to make more rational choices about their lifestyles. It is also possible the that the frequent blood tests required for the safety of clozapine treatment have the side benefit of keeping in touch with patients on a regular basis; this may improve the patients' engagement in treatment programs as well as enable closer monitoring and case management.

2.2. Comorbid Personality Disorders

Antisocial Personality Disorder and psychopathy are associated with criminal behavior, and schizophrenia patients with these comorbidities typically have a history of arrest and incarceration. When discharged into the community after a short stay in a psychiatric hospital, these patients are at a high risk for re-arrest or re-hospitalization. Their recidivistic criminal behavior results in a cycle of psychiatric admissions, discharges, arrests, and re-admissions or incarcerations.

Patients with these comorbid disorders are particularly difficult to treat. These personality disorders do not respond to any specific pharmacological interventions, and the usual psychiatric treatment programs are not effective. In response to the needs of this patient population, a specialized cognitive-behavioral treatment program has been developed (Kunz et al., 2004); (Yates et al., 2005). The program, called STAIR (System for Treatment and Abatement of Interpersonal Risk), aims to break the cycle of repeated hospitalization and incarceration. It is based at a State Hospital in New York City. The program teaches cognitive skills (problem solving, creative thinking, value enhancement, social skills, critical reasoning, and managing emotions). Skills are taught in group sessions; the program consists of 72 sessions. Furthermore, the STAIR incorporates a 12-step substance abuse program. Patients receive standard psychopharmacological treatment for their Axis I disorders (mostly psychosis). The first follow-up reports for 6-24 months after discharge are available for 85 patients; the results appear to support the effectiveness of the program (Kunz et al., 2004).

2.3. Treatment Non-Adherence

The cause or causes of non-adherence must be explored in individual patients. If the patient does not tolerate side effects, an effort must be made to reduce or eliminate them by adjusting the dose of antipsychotic, prescribing another medication to counteract the side effects (eg, an anticholinergic to reduce extrapyramidal symptoms), to switch to another antipsychotic, or to switch to a long-acting injectable antipsychotic. This has to be done in collaboration with the patient, and, if possible, with the patient's family. Therapeutic alliance based on mutual respect is conducive to psycho-education about acceptance of the illness, need to continue taking medication, and risks and benefits of treatments. Such psychosocial interventions are considered the first choice of treatment for patients demonstrating partial adherence to treatment (Kane, Leucht, Carpenter, and Docherty, 2003).

However, not all patients and their families are accessible to such efforts. The patients with comorbid substance abuse, those who have weak family and community support, the undomiciled, and the patients who simply refuse treatment are difficult to reach. Some of these patients have also comorbid personality disorders and a history of arrests and incarceration for violent crimes. Inpatient treatment for such patients was described in the preceding section. However, such treatment is not yet generally available. Thus, these patients are usually admitted or arrested after a violent incident, they are given antipsychotics, improve in several weeks, and they are discharged. Soon after the discharge, they discontinue their antipsychotic medication, do not keep their outpatient appointments, may start using drugs or alcohol, and become involved in violent incidents. Since such patients are repeatedly dangerous to others and themselves and are unable to break the cycle of violence, re-arrests and re-admissions, they may be subject to involuntary out-patient commitment (IOPC). Non-violent patients who are endangering only themselves may also qualify for IOPC.

IOPC is a legal intervention: a judge orders a patient residing in the community to adhere to recommended outpatient treatment. If the patient fails to do so, the responsible clinician may request the police to escort the patient to the treatment center. Once there, the clinicians try to persuade the patient to adhere to treatment, and evaluate him for inpatient commitment.

IOPC may have multiple positive effects beyond improving adherence to pharmacological treatments. It may also improve access to other treatments, result in better monitoring of patients' behavior and mental status, and thereby reduce the likelihood of a relapse. However, IOPC is coercive and may be seen as an infringement on the patients' civil liberties. Arguably, IOPC may not be necessary if appropriate voluntary treatment would be available in an adequately funded, well functioning mental health system. Such treatment might be expected to improve adherence through cooperation with the patient and his family. This libertarian argument has merit, but I think that there will always be patients who are just too difficult to reach on a voluntary basis even with an optimal mental health system. The question is, does IOPC yield better outcomes than voluntary outpatient treatment in difficult non-adherent patients?

A pilot study of IOPC in New York City suggested a negative answer to that question (Steadman et al., 2001). However, that study excluded patients with a history of violence, and the pick-up order procedures for non-adherent subjects were actually not implemented. A more definitive study was conducted in North Carolina (Swartz et al., 1999). Subjects who were hospitalized involuntarily were randomly assigned to IOPC or to voluntary outpatient treatment (control group) and followed up for 1 year. The control and IOPC groups did not differ significantly in readmission rates. However, a post-hoc analysis indicated that subjects with prolonged periods of IOPC (beyond that of the initial court order) had fewer readmissions and fewer hospital days than control subjects. (Swartz et al., 1999). The post-hoc nature of these analyses and various other methodological problems were criticized in subsequent correspondence (Segal, 2001; Szmukler and Hotopf, 2001). The North Carolina IOPC data were re-analyzed using violent behavior as the principal outcome variable. These analyses have demonstrated that IOPC of at least 6 months duration, combined with regular outpatient services, improved treatment adherence and reduced the risk of violent behavior and of substance abuse (Swanson et al., 2000). These important results await replication.

3. Psychopharmacology of Aggression in Schizophrenia

3.1. Current Treatments

Recent reviews have addressed various aspects of this topic (Citrome, Nolan, and Volavka, 2004; Citrome and Volavka, 2003; Citrome and Volavka, 2002b; Citrome and

Volavka, 2002a; Volavka, 2002). Therefore, there is no need for a detailed assessment of the field in this chapter.

Atypical Antipsychotics

Clozapine appeared to be the superior antipsychotic to treat hostility (Citrome et al., 2001) in 157 patients with schizophrenia or schizoaffective disorder participating in a randomized controlled trial comparing clozapine, olanzapine, riperidone, and haloperidol. Further analyses of measures of overt aggression in this trial (Volavka et al., 2004a) demonstrated that antipsychotic efficacy of clozapine was greatest in aggressive patients, whereas the opposite was true for risperidone and olanzapine. Importantly, a therapeutic dose of clozapine was necessary for the superior antiaggressive effect. This issue is particularly significant because it can take several weeks to titrate clozapine to a therapeutic dose. Therefore, it is important not to terminate a clozapine trial prematurely.

The results of that randomized controlled trial (Citrome et al., 2001; Volavka et al., 2004a)were consistent with a large number of preceding uncontrolled studies and case reports. The antiaggressive effect of clozapine appears to be independent of its sedative effect as well as of its general antipsychotic effect against positive symptoms of schizophrenia.

Risperidone demonstrated a selective effect on hostility that was superior to haloperidol (Czobor, Volavka, and Meibach, 1995). Similar antihostility/antiaggressive effects of risperidone were observed in a retrospective study of seclusion and restraint (Chengappa et al., 2000), but risperidone was not more effective than typical antipsychotics in other studies of aggression (Buckley et al., 1997; Beck et al., 1997). In a randomized double-blind trial, patients assigned to risperidone or olanzapine treatments were less likely to exhibit incidents of overt aggression than those on haloperidol (Volavka et al., 2004a). Effects of aripiprazole (Dillenschneider et al., 2004) and quetiapine (Chengappa, Goldstein, Greenwood, John, and Levine, 2003) on hostility and excitement were explored in post-hoc preliminary analyses and a case report (Citrome, Krakowski, Greenberg, Andrade, and Volavka, 2001).

Adjunctive Pharmacological Treatments

Adjunctive treatments that are added to an antipsychotic may have some antiaggressive effect. Adjunctive valproate was rated as the first-line treatment for aggressive behavior in schizophrenia patients in an expert consensus statement ((Kane et al., 2003), p.77). There is some evidence for the valproate efficacy in the first week of treatment treatment: In one study, 249 schizophrenia inpatients were randomly assigned to receive olanzapine plus placebo, olanzapine plus divalproex, risperidone plus placebo, or risperidone plus divalproex in a double-blind, 28-day trial. Adjunctive divalproex reduced hostility in the first week of treatment, but the efficacy was lost in the subsequent 3 weeks (Citrome et al., 2004). Efficacy in the initial stage of treatment is valuable since this is the time when much aggressive behavior occurs. However, as many as 30% of schizophrenia patients receive adjunctive valproate on a long-term basis, months beyond the initial stage of treatment (Citrome, Jaffe, and Levine, 2002). The antiaggressive or antihostility efficacy of such long-term valproate treatment has not been conclusively demonstrated in randomized clinical trials. Uncontrolled studies are reviewed elsewhere (Lindenmayer and Kotsaftis, 2000).

Adjunctive citalopram, a selective serotonin reuptake inhibitor, reduced aggressive behavior in chronic schizophrenia patients in a double-blind crossover study (Vartiainen et al., 1995).

Propranolol, a beta-adrenergic blocking agent, was first noted to reduce aggressive behavior in mice (Valzelli, Giacalone, and Garattini, 1967). Propranolol was then reported to reduce aggressive behavior following acute brain damage in humans (Elliott, 1977). It is possible (but not certain) that the antiaggressive effects of beta-blockers are mediated, at least in part, by adrenergic receptors. Propranolol has been used to control aggression primarily in patients with organic brain disease. However, there are some reports of propranolol added to antipsychotic regimens as an adjunctive treatment for schizophrenia (Yorkston et al., 1977; Sheppard, 1979); it reduced symptoms, including aggression. Case reports of successful treatment of aggression with propranolol in assaultive schizophrenic patients have been published (Sorgi, Ratey, and Polakoff, 1986; Whitman, Maier, and Eichelman, 1987). Reports of successful antiaggressive treatments with other beta-adrenergic blockers, such as nadolol, metoprolol, and pindolol, are summarized elsewhere (Volavka, 2002). The recent expert consensus guidelines list adjunctive beta blockers as a potential second line treatment for persistently aggressive schizophrenia patients ((Kane et al., 2003), p.77), but the treatment is not much used in clinical practice. Patients vary considerably in the degree to which they respond to beta blockers. Other adjunctive treatments tried as treatments of aggressive behavior in schizophrenia include lithium, carbamazepine, lamotrigine, and benzodiazepines.

Adjunctive Electroconvulsive Therapy (ECT)

Adjunctive ECT may be helpful in schizophrenia patients who are treatment-refractory, and in particular, in patients with persistent aggressive behavior. An open trial of ECT in combination with risperidone in male patients with schizophrenia and aggression resulted in a reduction in aggressive behavior for nine of the ten patients (Hirose, Ashby, Jr., and Mills, 2001). In that series of patients, bilateral ECT was administered five times a week, with a mean total number of 6.6 treatments. A large randomized clinical trial that will shed additional light on this issue is now in progress in the United States.

3.2. Future Directions

Tailoring treatments to fit individual aggressive patients is an important challenge for the future. Research into the phenotypic heterogeneity of assaults described in this chapter is a step towards this goal. The hypothesis that assaults (and perhaps patients) can be classified into aggression subtypes that respond to different treatments remains to be tested. The three subtypes that we isolated probably oversimplify and underestimate the real diversity of aggression.

The recently developed pharmacogenetic approaches to the treatments of mental illness can be expanded to address the problems of the heterogeneity of the aggressive behavior and its treatment. For example: As noted in the segment on beta-blockers above, there is a considerable variation in the patients' response to this treatment. Allelic variation of the COMT gene may underlie this variability. The Met allele of the COMT gene codes for the low activity form of this enzyme, resulting in an inadequate biotransformation of catecholamines. Theoretically, blocking beta-adrenergic transmission would partially correct for the relatively inadequate biotransformation of catecholamines. Therefore, one might test the hypothesis that the COMT allele coding for the low activity form of the enzyme will be associated with a greater antiaggressive effect of a beta-adrenergic blocking agent. If this is true, the patients most likely to benefit from beta-blocking agents would be the Met-Met homozygotes; the Val-Val homozygotes would be least likely to benefit. The observed interindividual variation of the response to beta-blockers would be explained, and the treatment could be tailored on the genetic basis.

There is a large group of persistently aggressive and criminal patients who are unlikely to benefit from any foreseeable biological treatment. Developing cognitive-behavioral or other similar programs for these patients is a major challenge for research and policy. Testing the effectiveness of such programs using established methods such as randomized clinical trials is usually not feasible due to political, ethical, and financial obstacles. It may be necessary to develop novel scientific methods for this important field. Somewhat similar obstacles are in the way of developing better methods for the reduction of comorbid substance abuse and improvement of treatment adherence.

References

Arseneault, L., Moffitt, T. E., Caspi, A., Taylor, P. J., and Silva, P. A. (2000). Mental disorders and violence in a total birth cohort: results from the Dunedin Study. *Arch.Gen.Psychiatry, 57,* 979-986.

Beck, N. C., Greenfield, S. R., Gotham, H., Menditto, A. A., Stuve, P., and Hemme, C. A. (1997). Risperidone in the management of violent, treatment-resistant schizophrenics hospitalized in a maximum security forensic facility. *Journal of the American Academy of Psychiatry and the Law, 25,* 461-468.

Bilder, R. M., Volavka, J., Lachman, H. M., and Grace, A. A. (2004). The Catechol-O-Methyltransferase Polymorphism: Relations to the Tonic-Phasic Dopamine Hypothesis and Neuropsychiatric Phenotypes. *Neuropsychopharmacology (In Press).*

Brennan, P. A., Mednick, S. A., and Hodgins, S. (2000). Major mental disorders and criminal violence in a Danish birth cohort. *Arch.Gen.Psychiatry, 57,* 494-500.

Buckley, P. F., Ibrahim, Z. Y., Singer, B., Orr, B., Donenwirth, K., and Brar, P. S. (1997). Aggression and schizophrenia: efficacy of risperidone. *J Am Psychiatry Law, 25,* 173-181.

Buckley, P. F., McCarthy, M., Chapman, P., Richman, C. G., and Yamamoto, B. (2000). Craving reduction and clozapine response in patients with comorbid substance abuse and schizophrenia. *Biological Psychiatry* 47, 18S-19S.

Chengappa, K. N., Goldstein, J. M., Greenwood, M., John, V., and Levine, J. (2003). A post hoc analysis of the impact on hostility and agitation of quetiapine and haloperidol among patients with schizophrenia. *Clin.Ther., 25,* 530-541.

Chengappa, K. N. R., Levine, J., Ulrich, R., Parepally, H., Brar, J., and Atzert, R. (2000). Impact of risperidone on seclusion and restraint at a state psychiatric hospital. 153rd

Annual Meeting of the American Psychiatric Association. New Research Abstracts, Chicago, IL , 199.

Citrome, L., Nolan, K. A., and Volavka, J. (2004). Science-Based Treatment of Aggression and Agitation. In D.Fishbein (Ed.), *The Science, Treatment, and Prevention of Antisocial Behaviors: Evidence-Based Practice* (1 ed., pp. 11-1-11-31). Kingston, NJ: Civic Research Institute, Inc.

Citrome, L., Casey, D. E., Daniel, D. G., Wozniak, P., Kochan, L. D., and Tracy, K. A. (2004). Adjunctive divalproex and hostility among patients with schizophrenia receiving olanzapine or risperidone. *Psychiatr.Serv., 55,* 290-294.

Citrome, L., Jaffe, A., and Levine, J. (2002). Datapoints - mood stabilizers: Utilization trends in patients diagnosed with schizophrenia 1994-2001. *Psychiatric Services, 53,* 1212.

Citrome, L., Krakowski, M., Greenberg, W. M., Andrade, E., and Volavka, J. (2001). Antiaggressive effect of quetiapine in a patient with schizoaffective disorder. *Journal of Clinical Psychiatry, 62,* 901.

Citrome, L. and Volavka, J. (2002a). Clinical management of persistent aggressive behavior in schizophrenia, Part I: Definitions, epidemiology, assessment, and acute treatment. *Essential Psychopharmacology, 5,* 1-16.

Citrome, L. and Volavka, J. (2002b). Clinical management of persistent aggressive behavior in schizophrenia, Part II: Long-term pharmacotherapeutic strategies. *Essential Psychopharmacology, 5,* 17-30.

Citrome, L. and Volavka, J. (2003). Treatment of Violent Behavior. In A.Tasman, J. Kay, and J. A. Lieberman (Eds.), *Psychiatry* (2 ed., pp. 2136-2146). Chichester: John Wiley and Sons, Ltd.

Citrome, L., Volavka, J., Czobor, P., Sheitman, B., Lindenmayer, J.-P., McEvoy, J. et al. (2001). Effects of clozapine, olanzapine, risperidone, and haloperidol on hostility in treatment-resistant patients with schizophrenia and schizoaffective disorder. *Psychiatric Services, 52,* 1510-1514.

Czobor, P., Volavka, J., and Meibach, R. C. (1995). Effect of risperidone on hostility in schizophrenia. *Journal of Clinical Psychopharmacology, 15,* 243-249.

Dillenschneider, A., Marcus, R., Kostic, D., Stringfellow, J., Hardy, S., Carson, W. et al. (2004). Short- and long-term effects of aripiprazole treatment on the excitement/hostility symptoms of schizophrenia. *The International Journal of Neuropsychopharmacology* 7, 243.

Dolder, C. R., Lacro, J. P., Dunn, L. B., and Jeste, D. V. (2002). Antipsychotic medication adherence: is there a difference between typical and atypical agents? *American Journal of Psychiatry, 159,* 103-108.

Drake, R. E., Xie, H., McHugo, G. J., and Green, A. I. (2000). The effects of clozapine on alcohol and drug use disorders among patients with schizophrenia. *Schizophr.Bull., 26,* 441-449.

Egan, M. F., Goldberg, T. E., Kolachana, B. S., Callicott, J. H., Mazzanti, C. M., Straub, R. E. et al. (2001). Effect of COMT Val108/158 Met genotype on frontal lobe function and risk for schizophrenia. *Proc.Natl.Acad.Sci.U.S.A, 98,* 6917-6922.

Elliott, F. A. (1977). Propranolol for the control of belligerent behavior following acute brain damage. *Annals of Neurology, 1,* 489-491.

Fernandes, C., Paya-Cano, J. L., Sluyter, F., D'Souza, U., Plomin, R., and Schalkwyk, L. C. (2004). Hippocampal gene expression profiling across eight mouse inbred strains: towards understanding the molecular basis for behaviour. *Eur.J Neurosci., 19,* 2576-2582.

Gogos, J. A., Morgan, M., Luine, V., Santha, M., Ogawa, S., Pfaff, D. et al. (1998). Catechol-O-methyltransferase-deficient mice exhibit sexually dimorphic changes in catecholamine levels and behavior. *Proceedings of the National Academy of Sciences of the United States of America, 95,* 9991-9996.

Green, A. I., Zimmet, S. V., Strous, R. D., and Schildkraut, J. J. (1999). Clozapine for comorbid substance use disorder and schizophrenia: do patients with schizophrenia have a reward-deficiency syndrome that can be ameliorated by clozapine? *Harv.Rev.Psychiatry, 6,* 287-296.

Hare, R. D. (1986). Twenty years of experience with the Cleckley psychopath. In W. H. Reid, D. Dorr, J. I. Walker, and J. W. I. Bonner (Eds.), *Unmasking the Psychopath. Antisocial Personality and Related Syndromes.* (pp. 3-27). New York: W. W. Norton and Company.

Hare, R. D. (1996). Psychopathy and antisocial personality disorder: a case of diagnostic confusion. *Psychiatric Times, February,* 39-40.

Hart, S. D., Hare, R. D., and Forth, A. E. (1994). Psychopathy as a risk marker for violence: development and validation of a screening version of the revised psychopathy checklist. In J. Monahan and H. J. Steadman (Eds.), *Violence and Mental Disorder. Developments in Risk Assessment* (pp. 81-98). Chicago: The University of Chicago Press.

Hirose, S., Ashby, C. R., Jr., and Mills, M. J. (2001). Effectiveness of ECT combined with risperidone against aggression in schizophrenia. *J.ECT., 17,* 22-26.

Jones, G., Zammit, S., Norton, N., Hamshere, M. L., Jones, S. J., Milham, C. et al. (2001). Aggressive behaviour in patients with schizophrenia is associated with catechol-O-methyltransferase genotype. *British Journal of Psychiatry, 179,* 351-355.

Kane, J. M., Leucht, S., Carpenter, D., and Docherty, J. P. (2003). The expert consensus guideline series. Optimizing pharmacologic treatment of psychotic disorders. *The Journal of Clinical Psychiatry, 64, Suppl. 12,* 1-100.

Kotler, M., Barak, P., Cohen, H., Averbuch, I. E., Grinshpoon, A., Gritsenko, I. et al. (1999). Homicidal behavior in schizophrenia associated with a genetic polymorphism determining low catechol O-methyltransferase (COMT) activity. *Am.J.Med.Genet., 88,* 628-633.

Kunz, M., Yates, K. F., Czobor, P., Rabinowitz, S., Lindenmayer, J. P., and Volavka, J. (2004). Course of patients with histories of aggression and crime after discharge from a cognitive-behavioral program. *Psychiatr.Serv., 55,* 654-659.

Lachman, H. M., Nolan, K. A., Mohr, P., Saito, T., and Volavka, J. (1998). Association between catechol O-methyltransferase genotype and violence in schizophrenia and schizoaffective disorder. *American Journal of Psychiatry, 155,* 835-837.

Lachman, H. M., Papolos, D. F., Saito, T., Yu, Y.-M., Szumlanski, C. L., and Weinshilboum, R. M. (1996). Human catechol-O-methyltransferase pharmacogenetics: description of a functional polymorphism and its potential application to neuropsychiatric disorders. *Pharmacogenetics, 6,* 243-250.

Lindenmayer, J.-P. and Kotsaftis, A. (2000). Use of sodium valproate in violent and aggressive behaviors: a critical review. *Journal of Clinical Psychiatry, 61,* 123-128.

Lindqvist, P. and Allebeck, P. (1990). Schizophrenia and assaultive behaviour: the role of alcohol and drug abuse. *Acta Psychiatrica Scandinavica, 82,* 191-195.

Mednick, S. A., Gabrielli, W. F., Jr., and Hutchings, B. (1983). Genetic influence in criminal behavior: evidence from an adoption cohort. In K.T.Van Dusen and S. A. Mednick (Eds.), *Prospective Studies of Crime and Delinquency* (pp. 39-56). Boston: Kluwer-Nijhoff Publishing.

Mednick, S. A., Gabrielli, W. F., Jr., and Hutchings, B. (1984). Genetic influences in criminal convictions: evidence from an adoption cohort. *Science, 224,* 891-894.

Mednick, S. A. and Kandel, E. (1988). Genetic and perinatal factors in violence. In T.E.Moffitt and S. A. Mednick (Eds.), *Biological Contributions to Crime Causation* (pp. 121-131). Dordrecht: Martinus Nijhoff Publishers.

Mednick, S. A., Pollock, V. E., Volavka, J., and Gabrielli, W. F., Jr. (1982). Biology and violence. In M.E.Wolfgang and N. A. Weiner (Eds.), *Criminal Violence* (4 ed., pp. 21-80). Beverly Hills: Sage Publications.

Mednick, S. A. and Volavka, J. (1980). Biology of crime. In N.Morris and M. Tonry (Eds.), *Crime and Justice: An Annual Review of Research* (pp. 85-158). Chicago: The University of Chicago Press.

Nolan, K. A., Czobor, P., Roy, B. B., Platt, M. M., Shope, C. B., Citrome, L. L. et al. (2003). Characteristics of assaultive behavior among psychiatric inpatients. *Psychiatr.Serv., 54,* 1012-1016.

Nolan, K. A., Volavka, J., Mohr, P., and Czobor, P. (1999). Psychopathy and violent behavior among patients with schizophrenia or schizoaffective disorder. *Psychiatric Services, 50,* 787-792.

Regier, D. A., Farmer, M. E., Rae, D. S., Locke, B. Z., Keith, S. J., Judd, L. L. et al. (1990). Comorbidity of mental disorders with alcohol and other drug abuse. Results from the Epidemiologic Catchment Area (ECA) Study. *JAMA, 264,* 2511-2518.

Rujescu, D., Giegling, I., Gietl, A., Hartmann, A. M., and Moller, H. J. (2003). A functional single nucleotide polymorphism (V158M) in the COMT gene is associated with aggressive personality traits. *Biol.Psychiatry, 54,* 34-39.

Segal, S. P. (2001). Effectiveness of involuntary outpatient commitment. *American Journal of Psychiatry, 158,* 654-656.

Sheppard, G. P. (1979). High-dose propranolol in schizophrenia. *British Journal of Psychiatry, 134,* 470-476.

Sorgi, P. J., Ratey, J. J., and Polakoff, S. (1986). Beta-adrenergic blockers for the control of aggressive behaviors in patients with chronic schizophrenia. *American Journal of Psychiatry, 143,* 775-776.

Steadman, H. J., Gounis, K., Dennis, D., Hopper, K., Roche, B., Swartz, M. et al. (2001). Assessing the New York City involuntary outpatient commitment pilot program. *Psychiatr.Serv., 52,* 330-336.

Strous, R. D., Bark, N., Parsia, S. S., Volavka, J., and Lachman, H. M. (1997). Analysis of a functional catechol O-methyltransferase gene polymorphism in schizophrenia: evidence for association with aggressive and antisocial behavior. *Psychiatry Research, 69,* 71-77.

Strous, R. D., Nolan, K. A., Lapidus, R., Diaz, L., Saito, T., and Lachman, H. M. (2003). Aggressive behavior in schizophrenia is associated with the low enzyme activity COMT polymorphism: A replication study. *Am.J.Med.Genet., 120B,* 29-34.

Swanson, J. W. (1994). Mental disorder, substance abuse, and community violence: an epidemiological approach. In J.Monahan and H. J. Steadman (Eds.), *Violence and Mental Disorder. Developments in Risk Assessment* (pp. 101-136). Chicago: The University of Chicago Press.

Swanson, J. W., Holzer, C. E., Ganju, V. K., and Jono, R. T. (1990). Violence and psychiatric disorder in the community: evidence from the Epidemiologic Catchment Area surveys. *Hospital and Community Psychiatry, 41,* 761-770.

Swanson, J. W., Swartz, M. S., Borum, R., Hiday, V. A., Wagner, H. R., and Burns, B. J. (2000). Involuntary out-patient commitment and reduction of violent behaviour in persons with severe mental illness . *Br.J.Psychiatry, 176,* 324-331.

Swartz, M. S., Swanson, J. W., Hiday, V. A., Borum, R., Wagner, H. R., and Burns, B. J. (1998a). Violence and severe mental illness: the effects of substance abuse and nonadherence to medication. *American Journal of Psychiatry, 155,* 226-231.

Swartz, M. S., Swanson, J. W., Hiday, V. A., Borum, R., Wagner, R., and Burns, B. J. (1998b). Taking the wrong drugs: the role of substance abuse and medication noncompliance in violence among severely mentally ill individuals. *Soc Psychiatry Psychiatr Epidemiol, 33 Suppl 1,* S75-S80.

Swartz, M. S., Swanson, J. W., Wagner, H. R., Burns, B. J., and Hiday, V. A. (2001). Effects of involuntary outpatient commitment and depot antipsychotics on treatment adherence in persons with severe mental illness. *J Nerv.Ment.Dis., 189,* 583-592.

Swartz, M. S., Swanson, J. W., Wagner, H. R., Burns, B. J., Hiday, V. A., and Borum, R. (1999). Can involuntary outpatient commitment reduce hospital recidivism?: Findings from a randomized trial with severely mentally ill individuals. *American Journal of Psychiatry, 156,* 1968-1975.

Szmukler, G. and Hotopf, M. (2001). Effectiveness of involuntary outpatient commitment. *American Journal of Psychiatry, 158,* 653-654.

Valzelli, L., Giacalone, E., and Garattini, S.¶□1967). Pharmacological control of aggressive behavior in mice. *European Journal of Pharmacology, 2,* 144-146.

Vartiainen, H., Tiihonen, J., Putkonen, A., Koponen, H., Virkkunen, M., Hakola, P. et al. (1995). Citalopram, a selective serotonin reuptake inhibitor, in the treatment of aggression in schizophrenia. *Acta Psychiatrica Scandinavica, 91,* 348-351.

Volavka, J. (2002). *Neurobiology of Violence*. (2 ed.) Washington, DC: American Psychiatric Publishing, Inc.

Volavka, J., Czobor, P., Nolan, K., Sheitman, B., Lindenmayer, J. P., Citrome, L. et al. (2004a). Overt aggression and psychotic symptoms in patients with schizophrenia treated with clozapine, olanzapine, risperidone, or haloperidol. *J Clin.Psychopharmacol., 24,* 225-228.

Volavka, J., Kennedy, J. L., Ni, X., Czobor, P., Nolan, K., Sheitman, B. et al. (2004b). COMT158 polymorphism and hostility. *Am J Med.Genet., 127B,* 28-29.

Whitman, J. R., Maier, G. J., and Eichelman, B. (1987). Beta-adrenergic blockers for aggressive behavior in schizophrenia [letter]. *American Journal of Psychiatry, 144,* 538-539.

Yates, K., Kunz, M., Czobor, P., Rabinowitz, S., Lindenmayer, J.P., Volavka, J. (2005) A cognitive, behaviorally based program for patients with persistent mental illness and a history of aggression, crime, or both: Structure and correlates of completers of the program. *J Am Acad Psychiatry Law,33:214-222.*

Yorkston, N. J., Zaki, S. A., Pitcher, D. R., Gruzelier, J. H., Hollander, D., and Sergeant, H. G. (1977). Propranolol as an adjunct to the treatment of schizophrenia. *Lancet, 2,* 575-578.

In: Adolescent Schizophrenia
Editors: J. T. Nillinghouse and R. P. Trotman

ISBN: 978-1-60692-370-2

Chapter VI

Body Image Deviation in Chronic Schizophrenia: A New Research

Reiko Koide and Akira Tamaoka
University of Tsukuba, Japan

Part I. Introduction

Schizophrenics' Body Image Aberration: An Overview

Since the time of Kraepelin (1919) and Bleuler (1911/1950), schizophrenics' deviant perceptions, feelings, and beliefs concerning their bodies have been described. In this section, the symptoms relevant to body image aberration that have been discussed for over the past half century, as well as psychological measures that were developed to understand these aberrations, are reviewed, to lead to the current status and future prospects for the study of the body image aberration in schizophrenia.

(1) Symptoms relevant To body image aberration

Disturbances of body experience in schizophrenic patients occur frequently. They have been observed as somatic delusions (McGlichrist and Cutting, 1995), coenaesthesis (Huber, 1957/1971; Rohricht and Priebe, 1997, Schmoll and Koch, 1989; Schmoll, 1994), disturbances of pain perception (Dworkin and Caligor, 1988; Rosenthal et al., 1990; Dworkin, 1994; Guieu et al., 1994; Lautenbacher and Krieg, 1994), out-of-body experiences (Blackmore, 1986; Twemlow et al., 1982), dysmorphophobia (Connolly and Gipson, 1978; Hay, 1983; Birtchnell, 1988; Snaith, 1992; Philips and McEloroy, 1993; deLeon et al., 1989; Phillips et al., 1994), and self-injury or self mutilation (Feldman, 1988; Burgess, 1991; Martin and Gattaz, 1991; Sonneburn and Vanstraelen, 1992 ; Weiser et al., 1993; Kennedy and Feldmann, 1994). In addition, the effects of body-oriented psychotherapy have been suggested (Darby, 1968; Berman, 1972).

According to Roehricht and Priebe (1997) in a report by Huber and Zerbin-Rueden (1979), although symptoms relevant to body distortion were seen in more than 74% of cases of schizophrenia, little attention has been paid to the evaluation of such symptoms. These symptoms are not included as a prominent component in psychometric approaches to measuring symptoms, such as the Brief Psychiatric Rating Scale, BPRS, (Overall and Gorham, 1962) or the Positive and Negative Symptoms Scale, PANSS (Kay et al., 1987). It is, however, not fair to regard that the issue as being rather neglected. Specifically, bizarre somatopsychic phenomena, e.g., feelings that the body is "being radiated," "being controlled by others," and "being cut up" have been reported in schizophrenia. Some of these abnormal body perceptions have been designated as "Schneiderian first rank symptoms" (Schneider, 1959/1976). Dysmorphophobia was relabeled as "one of the Somatoform Disorders" in 1980. "Body Dysmorphic Disorder," and its counterpart, "Delusional Disorder, Somatic Subtype" in 1987, were included in the *Diagnostic and Statistical Manual of Mental Disorders* (American Psychiatric Association, 1987), which produced considerable concern over delusions regarding appearance of the body (deLeon et al., 1989; Phillips et al., 1994). First, studies of these symptoms relevant to disturbances in body experiences in schizophrenia are reviewed to give an overview of how the problems have been described and treated.

Before Antipsychotics

Even in the era before antipsychotic agents, body image was rather attractive to those who studied the psychopathology of schizophrenia. Since Wernicke foreshadowed the idea of body image in his concept of "somatopsyche," this whole psychological field has been recognized as important in the understanding of psychotic patients, especially in relation to hallucinatory and delusional disturbances (Schilder, 1935; Angyal, 1936; Gerstmann, 1942; Bychowsky,1943).

The initial study of body image was a description of phantom limb. It was succeeded by neurological research from the 1910s to the 1950s (Head, 1911/1926; Pick, 1922; Schilder, 1935), and body image was conceived as the equivalent of "body schema" or "postural schema." This became the traditional definition of the concept. It was introduced to the field of psychiatry by Schilder (1935), and attempts were made to find similar distortions in psychiatric patients (Schilder, 1935; Angyal, 1936).

Bodily Hallucination and Somatic Delusion

Lukianowicz (1967) and McGlichrist and Cutting (1995) classified somatic delusions of psychotic cases including schizophrenia, showing that bodily delusions and hallucinations occur mostly inseparably. Bodily hallucination and somatic delusion have been treated as coenaesthesis in non-English speaking psychiatry, especially in Germany, where it was often reported to herald the onset of schizophrenia (Huber 1957,1971; Rohricht and Priebe, 1997; Schmoll and Koch, 1989; Schmoll, 1994).

Disturbances of Pain Perception

A disorder of proprioception in schizophrenic patients was earlier described by Rado (1959) as a basic element in schizophrenia. He speculated that extensive proprioceptive deficits could lead to distorted awareness of body image and eventually to the thought disorder characteristic of schizophrenia. Rosenbaum et al. (1965) and Ritzler and Rosenbaum (1974) conducted a series of experiments based on his theory with schizophrenic and non-schizophrenic subjects using weight discrimination as a measure of proprioception. They found that schizophrenics performed almost as well as normals do when asked to discriminate heavy weights, but did not discriminate light weights nearly as well as normals. Since light weights do not provide as much proprioceptive feedback as do heavy weights, these results were interpreted as demonstrating a proprioceptive deficit in the schizophrenics. These results, however, were not replicated by other authors (Ritzler, 1977; Leventhal et al., 1982), who showed that a proprioceptive deficit is not unique to schizophrenia.

Since the time of Kraepelin and Bleuler, "pain insensitivity" or "reduced sensitivity to pain" in schizophrenia has been documented. Kraepelin (1919) observed that patients with schizophrenia are often "less sensitive to bodily discomfort; they endure uncomfortable positions, pricks of a needle, injuries...burn themselves with their cigar, hurt themselves." Bleuler (1911/1950) noted that even in well-oriented patients one may often observe the presence of a complete analgesia which includes the deeper parts of the body as well as the skin. The patients "pluck out an eye, sit down on a hot stove and receive severe burns".

Although some authors reported that schizophrenic patients suffer headache (Varsamis and Adamson, 1976; Watson et al., 1981; Philips and Hunter, 1982; Torrey, 1989), the prevalence of pain complaints in schizophrenia appears to be lower than in other psychiatric disorders (Merskey, 1965; Spear, 1967; Delapaine et al., 1978; Watson et al., 1981). There are many descriptions of pain insensitivity in schizophrenia by surgeons and internists (Arieti, 1945; Marchand, 1959; West and Hecker, 1952; Vanderkampt, 1970; Apter, 1981, Fishbain 1982; Bickerstaff et al., 1988, Katz et al., 1990; Rosenthal et al., 1990). Dworkin (1994) reviewed the literature on this issue and argued that the insensitivity, although currently neglected, has important implications for physical health, self-mutilation, homelessness, premorbid development, and affective flattening in schizophrenic patients. Lautenbacher and Krieg (1994) also reviewed the literature and pointed out that pain insensitivity is important in elucidating pathophysiological mechanisms because pain perception is controlled by neurochemical and neurohormonal functions known to be affected by psychiatric disease processes. Guieu et al. (1994), however, assessed the pain thresholds of ten schizophrenic patients and ten controls by measuring the leg flexion nociceptive reflex threshold, and concluded that in most cases the increase in pain threshold is the result of attitude and not alterations in brain function.

Out-of-Body Experiences

A number of studies have pointed out the confusion in the existing psychiatric literature concerning the status of consciousness in which there is an altered perception of the mind/body relationship. They defined out-of-body experience (OBE) as an altered state of consciousness in which one's mind or awareness is experienced as separated from one's physical body. They argued that the increasing numbers of patients who are involved in such phenomena, traditionally classified as psychopathological, should not be treated in the way that a symptom is usually treated (e.g., interpretation or medication) but should be viewed by a physician with "benign neglect" (Twemlow, et al., 1982).

Gabbard et al. developed a questionnaire, Profile of Out-of-Body Experiences, POBE, that included 51 items based on reports of near-death experiences, mystical-religious literature, and philosophical-occult-psychotic literature describing OBE experiences. They tried to clarify this group of phenomena by differentiating OBE from depersonalization, autoscopic phenomena, and schizophrenic body distortions (such as boundary loss). They selected seven points to differentiate OBE from the disturbances in corporal perception found in schizophrenia. That is, the bodily distortions in schizophrenic patients are characterized by loss of reality testing, chronic difficulty with delineation of body boundaries, varied bodily distortions, being uncertain of the location of the body, profound regression in personality, blurred identity, and being experienced as "going crazy," whereas those experiencing OBE show intact reality testing, have episodic and short-lived experiences, basically unvaried distortion, are certain of their location, show no evidence of regression, have an intact identity, and are not experienced as "going crazy."

Blackmore (1986) administered POBE to schizophrenic patients, along with two other questionnaires to assess perception and symptoms, and showed that there is no evidence to consider the typical OBE as pathological or as symptomatic of schizophrenia.

Dysmorphophobia

Extreme concern with aspects of personal appearance was called dysmorphophobia by Morselli in 1886 (Birtchnell, 1988; Phillips, 1991), who defined it as "a subjective feeling of ugliness or physical defect that the patient feels is noticeable to others, although his appearance is within normal limits." Despite its relative neglect in American psychiatry, it is now termed "Somatoform Disorder" in DSM III (1980), "Body Dysmorphic Disorder (BDD)" in DSM III-R with its counterpart, "Delusional Disorder, Somatic Subtype (DDSS)" (1987). It is a distressing and impairing disorder that may lead to occupational and social dysfunction as well as unnecessary and costly cosmetic surgery and dermatologic treatment (Phillips, 1991), and an increase in this disorder has been reported (Phillips et al., 1993; Hollander et al., 1993). It is still described with the term BDD under the heading of Somatoform Disorder in DSM-IV (1994).

In the 19th century, the term "dysmorphophobia" described those patients who present with "a fear of being misshapen" when in fact objectively they have no cause for complaint. However, numerous reports of dysmorphophobia in psychiatric morbidity, including schizophrenia, have been reported (Connolly and Gipson, 1978; Edgerton et al., 1960; Jacobsen et al., 1960; Hay, 1970). In the 1980s, there were continuing debates as to its status as a symptom or discrete psychiatric illness; that is, it is not a phobia because there is no fear of physical abnormality per se—the ugliness of others is tolerated. It was remarked that dysmorphophobia is non-specific as a symptom and can occur in a variety of different psychiatric syndromes, from a sensitive personality development to an attenuated schizophrenic illness (Hay, 1970/1983).

In the 1940s to the 1960s, psychodynamic theories attempted to recognize that a complaint about appearance might be understood in terms of psychological defense mechanisms (Meyer et al., 1960; Jacobsen et al., 1960; Linn and Goldman, 1949; Hill and Silver, 1950). Body parts took on a psychological significance and symbolic function, and a complaint might reflect an underlying conflict. However, reports of excellent results from surgery on the minimally deformed led to criticism to these theories, suggesting neurotic, and even psychotic, patients can benefit from cosmetic surgery (Edgerton et al., 1960; Hay, 1973).

Although the original definition of dysmorphophobia states that the appearance is within normal limits, diagnostic criteria proposed for dysmorphophobia allow for a slight physical anomaly to be present, but with the patient's concern judged disproportionately great (Andreasen and Bardach, 1977). Birtchnell (1988) regarded it as important to maintain a distinction between those patients with minimal deformity (the normal but less than attractive) who might considerably benefit from surgery and those with primary dysmorphophobia distinguished by the vagueness of the complaint, e.g., "the skin under my eyes joins my nose in a funny way," where surgery is contraindicated, rather than, for example, "the tip of my nose is rather bulbous."

The disorder once termed dysmorphophobia was renamed body dysmorphic disorder (BDD) in DSM III-R. As Snaith (1992) reviewed, DSM III-R considered the disorder under two headings: (1) delusional disorder, somatic type, and (2) body dysmorphic disorder. The distinctions between these two categories rests on whether the bodily concern has the characteristics of a true delusion, but a clear distinction cannot always be made. DSM III-R differentiated BDD, a nonpsychotic somatoform disorder in which insight is present, from its delusional counterpart, a psychotic disorder in which insight is absent. The delusional variant of BDD was reported as a more severe form of the disorder (Phillips et al., 1994).

Self-Injury or Self Mutilation

Self-injurious behaviour of various sorts occurs in an appreciable number of individuals with schizophrenia, as well as in those with other disorders (Burgess, 1991). Self-mutilation has been defined as "painful , destructive and injurious acts upon the body without the apparent intent to commit suicide" (Pattison and Kahan, 1983). Reports of self-mutilation in patients with schizophrenia include descriptions of unilateral and bilateral eye enucleation (Feldman, 1988; Kennedy and Feldmann, 1994), self-laceration (Shore et al., 1978; Sweeny and Zamecnik, 1981), and self-amputation of various parts of the body, including the hand (Schweitzer, 1990), breast (Coons et al., 1986), ear (Silva, et al., 1989; Weiser et al., 1993), penis and testicles (Schweitzer, 1990; Martin and Gattaz, 1991), and in what is arguably the most extreme case reported to date, virtually the entire face (Scheftel et al., 1986).

Burgess (1991) studied the relationship of depression and cognitive impairment to self-injury in psychiatric patients including schizophrenics, showing that self-injury was correlated with neurocognitive deficits in borderline and schizophrenic groups.

Body-Oriented Psychotherapy

An early theoretical assumption, currently recognized as invalid, was that the core disturbance in schizophrenia is a breakdown of ego boundaries leading to a dedifferentiation of the self from the non-self (Federn, 1952; Freeman et al., 1958). According to this theory, what is sensed as thought (a process occurring within the mental and physical boundary) is no longer distinguished from what is sensed as lying outside the ego boundary (Berman, 1972). Psychoanalytic theorists have stressed the important role the individual's body plays in bringing about the formation of the ego (e.g., Federn, 1952; Fenichel, 1954; Ferenczi, 1926; Freud, 1962), and the maintenance of the distinction between ego and non-ego was a controversial issue for psychotherapeutic treatment of schizophrenia.

Des Lauriers (1962) theorized that the recovery process in schizophrenia could be conceptualized as a progressive definition and demarcation of the schizophrenic's ego boundaries through a systematically increased awareness of body limits and bodily self. In order to accomplish this, the psychotherapist attempted to stimulate in the schizophrenic patient awareness of, and interest in, the bodily self as the separating boundary from that which is not himself (Darby, 1968; Des Lauriers, 1962). Studies conducted with an inkblot boundary index developed by Fisher and Cleveland (1958), the Barrier and Penetration scores, lend some support to the above conception of schizophrenia and the recovery process, in that schizophrenics were differentiated from neurotics and normals on the basis of their lower Barrier and higher Penetration scores (Fisher and Cleveland, 1958; Reitman and Cleveland, 1964; Holtzman et al., 1961) and that as a schizophrenic improved clinically, his Penetration scores decreased (Cleveland, 1960a). Fisher and Cleveland (1968) suggested that special treatment efforts, aimed at re-identifying and redefining bodily limits, should improve these patients. Because a question arises as to whether directly focusing the schizophrenic patient's awareness and attention on his own body can effect a redefinition of boundaries, attempts were made to demonstrate that focusing on somatic stimuli leads to subsequent changes in inkblot boundary indexes, implying, at least, that it can (Fisher and Renik, 1966; Renik and Fisher, 1968). Attempts were also made to expect alteration of body image change in these indexes by inducing somatic awareness in groups of hospitalized schizophrenics (Darby, 1968). Quinlan and Harrow (1974) examined the boundary in a sample of acute schizophrenics by the use of four types of Rorschach indexes including Barrier and Penetration scores. Their results support the hypothesis that schizophrenics give certain types of responses considered indicative of boundary disturbance, such as contamination responses, although Barrier and Penetration indexes are more benign signs of boundary diffusion.

(2) Psychological Measurement of Body Image Aberration

The above observations have led to an assumption that body image aberration or deviation exists in schizophrenia, and that it is related to the core of schizophrenia. Attempts were made, using the Rorschach test (Quinlan and Harrow 1974; Fisher and Cleveland, 1958/1968; Fisher, 1963), Drawing test (Kokonis, 1972) and inquiries (Fisher and Seidner, 1963; Chapman et al., 1978; Coleman et al., 1996; Koide, 1985; Oosthuizen et al., 1998), to point to characteristic deviations of body image in schizophrenic patients. These are the Body Distortion Questionnaire, BDQ, (Rohricht and Priebe, 1996), the Perceptual Aberration Scale, PAS, (Coleman et al., 1996; Chapman et al., 1978), Dysmorphic Concern Questionnaire, DCQ (Oosthuizen et al., 1998), and the present Body Image Questionnaire, BIQ (Koide, 1985). However, none of these measures are regarded as well-established (Rohricht and Prieb, 1997).

Projective Method

Early attempts to measeure body image aberrations were made through indirect means, that is, projective techniques. Figure-drawing techniques (Goodenough, 1928; Machover, 1949), have been used often by researchers (Cancro, 1971; Jasker and Reed, 1963; Sugarman and Cancro, 1964); however, most of the differences between schizophrenic and normal subjects appear to reflect nothing more than general inadequacy of drawing skill by schizophrenics (Swensen, 1957/1968). Barrier and penetration percepts on the Rorschach Test were inferred from body image (Fisher and Cleveland, 1958/1968). Barrier percepts are ones that emphasize peripheral-boundary-defining qualities of the percepts (e.g., flower pot or knife in armor). Penetration percepts involve penetration of outer surfaces of things (e.g., squashed bug or x-ray picture). Lowered barrier scores and heightened penetration scores have been reported in schizophrenia (Fisher and Cleveland, 1958/1968; Reitman and Cleveland, 1964; Holtzman et al., 1961/64). A lack of difference has also been reported (Jasker and Reed, 1963). While support for schizophrenic deviancy on the barrier and penetration scores is strong, acceptance of such evidence as support for schizophrenic body-image aberration requires belief in the projective hypothesis (Chapman et al., 1978).

Experimental Measurement

More direct attempts were made to measure body image aberration in the laboratory setting. Traub et al. (1967) performed an experiment in which the subjects adjust a body-distorting mirror until they believe that it reflects them accurately, with the result that schizophrenic patients erred more than the normal control subjects. Controversial results were presented in studies in which the patients were asked to judge the size of their own body. Cleveland (1960) and Cleveland et al. (1962) reported that schizophrenics overestimate the size of their various body parts (hand, foot, stomach, heart) more than control subjects do, although Weckowicz and Sommer (1960) found that schizophrenics underestimate sizes of their hands and feet. Dillon (1962) and Fisher (1966) found no difference between schizophrenic and normal subjects.

Questionnaire Measurement

The first questionnaire that attempted to measure body image aberration in schizophrenia is the Body Experience Questionnaire, BEQ, which is a true-false questionnaire developed by Fisher and Seidner (1963) and Fisher (1964). Their findings showed greater body image aberration in schizophrenics than in non-schizophrenic subjects, but their BEQ focused to a large extent on hypochondriacal concerns and feelings of body inadequacy rather than the more extreme psychosis-like deviancy of perception of the body that is usually attributed to schizophrenia.

Chapman et al. (1978) developed another questionnaire to measure schizophrenic body image aberration, the Perceptual Aberration Scale, PAS, which is composed of 28 items and a four-point rating sale. Items were intended to tap five kinds of deviant experiences that are uncommon in normal people. The experiences dealt with (a) unclear boundaries of the body, (b) feeling of unreality of, or estrangement from, parts of the body, (c) a sense of deterioration of the body, (d) perceptions of change in size, relative proportions, or spatial relationships of body parts, and (e) changes in the appearance of the body. The scale was standardized on normal control groups. Male schizophrenics reported more body image aberration than normal control subjects, but only a portion of the schizophrenics were deviant. In addition, schizophrenic body image aberrations were negatively correlated with time since first hospitalization and had no correlation with the Physical Anhedonia Scale (Chapman et al., 1976) for schizophrenia, suggesting that the two scales, PAS and Physical Anhedonia Scale, may identify alternative manifestations of proneness toward the same schizophrenia, that is, schizophrenia and schizophrenia-proneness. Coleman et al. (1996) administered PAS to a sample of 2000 students to detect a group of schizotypy in a study conducted to examine the empirical links between schizophrenia and schizotypic psychopathology. Through comparisons of thought disorder assessed by the Thought Disorder Index, TDI (Coleman et al., 1993), between high and low PAS groups, the authors supported the hypothesis that psychometrically identified schizotypic individuals tapped by PAS display thought disorder similar to that of schizophrenia.

Oosthuizen et al. (1998) developed a four-point questionnaire, the Dysmorphic Concern Questionnaire, DCQ, to assess dysmorphic concerns, and tried to establish a correlation with clinical variables. The DCQ was loosely based on the General Health Questionnaire, GHQ. A series of seven statements was devised, based on the dysmorphic concern literature, to capture the essence of the problem (e.g., concern about physical appearance, considering oneself misshapen) and past attempts to deal with the problem (e.g., consulting a plastic surgeon, covering up supposed defects). The DCQ was administered to 63 patients including 33 schizophrenics. The results showed dysmorphic concern is often a reflection of cognitive set rather than a diagnosis itself.

The Body Image Questionnaire, BIQ, is a seven-step self-rating questionnaire with 59 body referring items, especially devised to measure schizophrenic body image deviation (Koide, 1985). The BIQ was developed on the basis of the clinical observations made through contact with chronic schizophrenic patients by clinicians and the attempts to grasp their deviations through assessing rather persistent attitudes or feelings toward the patients' own bodies, which are measurable on a graded continuum with those of normals. Thus, what is assessed by the BIQ is not a psychosis-like body distortion experience itself but an underlying readiness for observable aberrant behaviors including distorted body experiences. The patients' deviated concern about their body is revealed by observations. A middle-aged female schizophrenic patient tried to eat her glasses to exemplify the strength of her teeth (image of strong teeth). A young male patient continued to reject walking outside the hospital in the treatment programs because he felt tight like a stone when he tried to go out (image of tightness caused by relaxation). One young female patient talked about her wish to commit suicide because, she said, she wanted to avoid situations in which she imagined herself unable to move her own body by herself (image of becoming immobile). The items of the BIQ were arranged to include three prospectively hypothetical components: namely, anatomical, functional and other psychological elements such as mood and primitive sensation.

Objective of the Study

A wide variety of studies has appeared on body image aberration in schizophrenia; however, the problem inherent in schizophrenic body image aberration remains elusive.

Earlier, the body image problems in schizophrenia were regarded as something related to psychotic symptoms, particularly with delusion and hallucination. Our perceptions of the schizophrenia have changed dramatically, particularly over the past two decades. During 1980s, the predominant view of the phenomenology of schizophrenia broadened beyond a narrow focus on psychotic symptoms to include negative symptoms, proprioceptive deficits, and self-injury representing body image problems. In the 1990s, another fundamental change in our perception of the disorder occurred. With this change, we have expanded the phenomenology of schizophrenia even further, beyond symptoms altogether, to include a strong emphasis on neurocognitive aspects of schizophrenia (Green and Neuchterlein, 1999).

Schizophrenia has consequently been investigated using "neuropsychological" procedures in order to uncover evidence of discrete neurological damage or dysfunction that may account for the great impairments in judgment, attention, concentration, planning ability and anticipation. In the late 1970s, a new era of neuropsychological study of schizophrenia began with three different review articles in which the low performance on neuropsychological test in functional patients was compared to organic patients (Goldstein, 1978; Heaton et al., 1978; Malec, 1978), and with the initial publication of in vivo evidence of ventricular enlargement in schizophrenia, as revealed by computerized tomography (CT) (Johonstone et al., 1976; Weinberger et al., 1979).

Focus has been on clarifying the relationships between neurocognitive deficits and psychotic symptoms (Cornblatt et al., 1985; Green and Walker, 1985; Neuchterlein et al., 1986; Green et al., 1992) and negative symptoms (Neuchterlein et al., 1986; Censits et al., 1997; Buchanan et al., 1997), between neurocognitive deficits and functional outcome (Green, 1996), between neurocognitive deficits and insight (Silverstein and Zerwic, 1985; Young et al., 1993; Lysaker and Bell, 1994; Cuesta and Peralta, 1994) and social cognition (Schneider et al., 1995; Bryson et al., 1997). In a current overview, Green and Nuechterlein (1999) searched for meaningful psychopharmacological and cognitive/behavioral interventions for neurocognitive deficits in schiziophrenia. Conventional antipsychotic agents are generally effective for psychotic symptoms, but their effects on neurocognition are relatively weak (Cassens et al., 1990; Strauss, 1993). Novel antipsychotic medications are more encouraging (Hagger et al., 1993; Green et al., 1997; Jeste et al., 1998; Keefe et al., 1999; Kern et al., 1999; Meltzer and McGurk, 1999). Conventional antipsychotic medications involve much coadministration of anticholinergic medications (e.g., benoztropine mesylate) that are known to have a negative effect on neurocognition (Spohn and Strauss, 1989).

To consider body image aberration in the above context, which deficit of body image comes from symptoms and which from medication should be clarified first. The questions are (1) Is body image aberration a result of symptoms seen in attenuated schizophrenic illness? (2) Is body image aberration an effect of medications? (3) What is the schizophrenics' body image's inherently aberrational part? Is there any intact part? (4) Is it remediable by behavioral/cognitive or psychopharmacological intervention? A full investigation of these basic questions is now required. Each section in this chapter is the attempt to clarify these basic problems.

Part II. Studies Using Body Image Questionnaire (BIQ)

Study 1. Body image aberration and clinical characteristics

Introduction

In the era of pre-antipsychotics, disturbance of body experiences in schizophrenia had been documented as pathological experiences, especially in relation to hallucinatory and delusional disturbances. Since the 1970s, several concepts about the course of schizophrenia and recovery from it have been developed in the search for new perspectives (Strauss 1989; Harding et al., 1992). Because there is a growing interest in the recovery phase of schizophrenia, their body image characteristics should be refocused as multi-phased deviation from the normal experiences. In this context, the body image should be redefined rather comprehensively as persistent attitudes and feelings toward one's own body, which would preserve deleterious as well as ameliorative effects in the illness-environment interaction of disorder and recovery. In addition, with the availability of neuroleptics since mid. 1950s, undesirable physical reactions caused by drugs may also contribute to negative body image.

The aim of the study in this section was to reexamine the body image distortion perceived by schizophrenics, using the Body Image Questionnaire, BIQ, (Koide,1982/1985). Special inquiries were made concerning the influence of the clinical variables such as positive and negative symptoms, insight and neuroleptic dosage on body image aberration. The questions addressed in this sections are (1) What are the components of body images? (2) Which phases of body image are aberrant in schizophrenia? (3) Which aberrant body images are related to symptoms? (4) Which aberrant body images are associated with favorable signs of remission? (5) Is body image aberration related to neuroleptic dosage?

Method

Assessment of Body Image Deviation

Body image was assessed using the BIQ, a seven-step self-rating scale (scored as 1 to 7) with three hypothetical components, anatomical, functional and psychological. (See Appendix 1.)

Assessment of Clinical Characteristics

Positive symptoms were assessed using the Scale for Assessment of Positive Symptoms, SAPS, (Andreasen, 1983). Negative symptoms were assessed using the Scale for Assessment of Negative Symptoms, SANS, (Andreasen, 1981). Insight was assessed through Schedule for Assessing Insight, SAI, which comprises three main component scores that include acceptance, recognition of illness, and relabeling of pathological experiences, and one supplemental component, i.e., the hypothetical contradiction, which measures amenability to delusional experiences (David, 1990).

Subjects

The study sample consisted of 93 chronic schizophrenics; 44 were men and 49 were women. The mean (SD) age of the patients was 48.5 (10.1) years. All of them were inpatients at chronic psychiatric wards of a mental hospital in Ibaraki Prefecture in Japan. They were diagnosed as schizophrenic, on the basis of medical records, according to DSM-IV criteria (Subtypes: 24 Paranoid types, 40 Disorganized types, 25 Residual types, 4 Undifferentiated types). The mean (SD) duration of hospitalization was 24.1 (10.6) years, and the mean (SD) age of onset was 24.0 (7.0) years old. Their mean (SD) dose of neuroleptics was 469.8 (397.5) mg/day of chlorpromazine equivalent dose. The mean SAPS scores of the subjects was 26.2. The mean of SANS scores was 67.8. The mean SAI score was 8.4. The normal control group was comprised of 177 normally functioning adults of whom 78 were men and 99 were women. The mean (SD) age was 44.9 (12.6) years old. The normal adults were attending university summer school classes in psychology, and were confirmed to be normal by the General Health Questionnaire, the GHQ (short form, Goldberg, 1972; Goldberg and Williams, 1988). All subjects were informed of the purpose of the study and actively participated with written informed consent. (See Table 1.)

Table 1. Demographic and clinical characteristics of subjects. (Studies 1 and 5.)

	Schizophrenic (N=93)	Normal (N=177)
Demographic characteristics		
Mean Age	48.5	44.9
Gender (% male)	47.3	44.1
Clinical characteristics	Mean (Range)	
Age of Onset	24.0 (14-45)	
Years of Hospitalization	24.1 (3-47)	
Dose of CPZ (mg/day)	469.8 (30-2156)	
SAPS	26.2 (0-94)	
SANS	67.8 (9-152)	
SDS	42.5 (24-64)	
SAI (Insight)	8.4 (0-14)	

Data Analysis

Comparisons of Means of each BIQ Item Scores

The means of the scores of 59 BIQ items were compared between schizophrenic and normal control groups using t-test.

Factor Analysis of the Body Image Questionnaire

On the bases of tentative preliminary analysis, 32 out of the original 59 items that proved to be not relevant to the factor analysis were excluded. However, two exceptional functional items (items 37, 41) from the excluded non-contributing items that proved to be important for discrimination when each item score was compared were re-included. The items of the final version pertain to smallness (items 8, 40, 54, 55), fatness (items 15, 28, 56) and roundness (items 24, 52) for the anatomical body image component; difficulty in manipulating his/her own body into action (items 9, 13, 21), lack of strength (items 1, 3), unusual concern over digestive functions (items 38, 53) and exceptional criterion-oriented standards (items 37, 41) for the functional component; and dissatisfaction and ugliness (items 10, 12, 27, 32), lack of vitality (items 31, 59) and fragility (items 19, 26, 39) for the psychological component.

Table 2. Means of BIQ items differentiating diagnostic groups. (Study 1.)

	Schizophrenic	Normal
01. My body is weak.	3.913	3.175***
03. I often get sick.	3.774	2.943***
06. My body is underdeveloped.	3.612	3.176**
07. My body is clean. ®	3.065	2.604**
09. I move slowly	4.193	3.649**
13. I am good at athletics.®	4.301	3.556**
17. I often lose my balance.	3.591	3.153*
19. I am often injured.	4.010	3.508**
23. My mood is numb.	4.279	3.875*
25. I am clumsy with my hands.	4.064	3.593*
26. I seldom catch a cold. ®	4.173	3.519**
29. My voice is feeble.	4.011	3.491**
31. I am always cheerful. ®	3.752	3.255**
37. I can work well in dark rooms. ®	5.258	4.429***
39. My body is susceptible to infection.	3.892	3.278**
41. I cannot move my body freely.	3.239	2.858*
42. My heart is strong. ®	3.397	2.949*
43. I don’t mind being touched by others. ®	4.591	4.000**
44. My body is not meager. ®.	3.709	3.339*
45. I seldom get excited.	4.043	3.653*
47. My teeth are weak.	4.826	4.079***
55. My arms are unusually long. ®	3.989	3.680*
59. I always feel energetic.®	3.957	3.491**

*P<0.05, **P<0.01, ***P<0.001.

The combined (schizophrenic and normal) data of the three BIQ hypothetical components, viz., anatomical, functional and psychological, were separately factor-analyzed using varimax rotation as the principal method, and the means of the factor scores were compared between the schizophrenic and normal control groups using *t*-tests. The factors that proved to be significant in differentiating schizophrenic and normal groups were compared further between the schizophrenic subgroups using *t*-tests. The schizophrenic subgroups were compared according to high (above or equal to mean) and low (lower than mean) scores on subscales and total scores of SAPS, SANS and SAI. Sub-grouping was also done according to the clinical factors of years of hospitalization and age at onset of disease, as well as daily equivalent dose of chlorpromazine. The SPSS (version 10) was used for statistical analysis.

Results

Group Differences of the BIQ Item Scores

The 23 out of 59 BIQ items proved to be differentiating two diagnostic groups. They were being weak, being prone to sickness, being underdeveloped, being dirty, moving slowly, being poor at athletics, being prone to losing balance, being prone to injury, being numb, being clumsy with hands, being prone to catching colds, speaking with a feeble voice, being always gloomy, being unable to work in dark rooms, being susceptible to infection, being unable to move his/her body freely, having a weak heart, minding being touched by others, being meager, not being prone to becoming excited, having weak teeth, having unusually long arms and being listless. (See Table 2.)

Factor Analysis and Obtained Differential Factors

Factor Analyses

Factor analyses of the three BIQ components, anatomical, functional, and psychological, using varimax rotation as the principal method, identified three factors with eigenvalues greater than 1 for each component. All items except two (items 37 and 41) had substantial loading on each of the factors. Total variances explained were 47.15%, 52.16% and 44.96%, respectively. Each of the three anatomical factors was composed of items indicating the images of smallness, fatness and roundness, respectively. Each of the three functional factors was composed of items indicating the images of dullness in movement, powerlessness and unusually strong gastrointestinal function, respectively. Each of the three psychological factors was composed of items indicating the images of dissatisfaction, lifelessness and fragility, respectively. (See Table 3 and 4.)

Differentiating factors

Based on the results of the *t*-test of means of obtained factor scores of schizophrenic and normal control groups, five proved to be factors that differentiated the two groups. These factors are F-1 (dullness in movement, t=3.099, df=159.101, p=0.002), F-2 (powerlessness, t=4.458, df=136.065, p=0.000), F-3 (unusually strong gastrointestinal function, t=2.332, df=263, p=0.020), P-2 (lifelessness, t=3.042,df=260, p=0.003) and P-3 (fragility, t=4.507, df=260, p=0.000). (See Table 4.)

Related Clinical Characteristics

Symptoms

The results of the *t*-test of differentiating factor scores between schizophrenic subgroups composed of SAPS and SANS scores are shown in Table 5. The high-score (>5.28) group on hallucinations (SAPS-1) showed a statistically significantly higher factor score on F-2 (powerlessness, t=2.567, df=89, p=0.012) and P-2 (lifelessness, t=2.426, df=89, p=0.017) than the low-score group. The high-score (>10.12) group on delusions (SAPS-2) showed a statistically significantly higher factor score on F-2 (powerlessness, t=2.100, df=89, p=0.039) and P-2 (lifelessness, t=3.814, df=89, p=0.000) than the low-score group. The high-score (>8.96) group on positive formal thought disorder (SAPS-4) showed a statistically significantly higher factor score on F-2 (powerlessness, t=2.819, df=89, p=0.006) than the low-score group. The high-score (>26.2) group on total SAPS showed a statistically significantly higher factor score on F-2 (powerlessness, t=2.358, df=89, p=0.021) and P-2 (lifelessness, t=2.175, df=89, p=0.032) than the low-score group.

Table 3. Factor structure of BIQ. (Study 1.)

Items of BIQ components	Factors and Factor Loadings			h^2
Anatomical	*A-1*	*A-2*	*A-3*	
55. My arms are short.	0.716			0.539
08. I am short.	0.65			0.463
54. My legs are short.	0.636			0.418
40. My hands are small.	0.457			0.239
28. I am fat.		0.796		0.673
15. My body is not skinny.		0.792		0.629
56. My neck is short.		0.437		0.348
24. My body is not rough.			0.731	0.536
52. My body is round.			0.413	0.401
Functional	*F-1*	*F-2*	*F-3*	
13. I am poor at athletics.	0.808			0.654
09. I move slowly	0.783			0.644
21. I walk slowly.	0.693			0.492
37. I cannot work well in dark rooms.				0.027
03. I often get sick.		0.881		0.804
01. My body is weak.		0.802		0.693
41. I cannot move my body freely.				0.250
38. My stomach is unusually strong.			0.812	0.666
53. My bowels are unusually strong.			0.673	0.462
Psychological	*P-1*	*P-2*	*P-3*	
32. My body is unattractive.	0.693			0.535
27. I am satisfied with my body.	0.684			0.487
12. My body is ugly.	0.671			0.476

Table 3. (Continued)

Items of BIQ components	Factors and Factor Loadings			h^2
10. My body is defective.	0.568			0.385
59. I always feel listless.		0.933		0.903
31. I am always gloomy.		0.506		0.290
26. I often catch colds.			0.586	0.352
39. My body is susceptible to infection.			0.554	0.339
19. I am often injured.			0.496	0.279

Note: Only items that loaded at >.400 are shown.

Table 4. Means of factor scores in schizophrenic and control groups. (Study 1.)

Anatomical Factors	Schizophrenic	Control
A-1. Smallness	0.092	-0.047
A-2. Fatness	0.114	-0.058
A-3. Roundness	0.057	0.029
Functional Factors		
F-1. Dullness in movement	0.246	-0.128**
F-2. Powerlessness	0.373	-0.195**
F-3. Unusually strong gastrointestinal function	0.168	-0.088*
Psychological Factors	Schizophrenic	Control
P-1. Dissatisfaction	0.003	-0.018
P-2. Lifelessness	0.239	-0.127**
P-3. Fragility	0.278	-0.147**

*p<0.05, **p<0.01.

The high-score (>12.2) group on avolition-apathy (SANS-3) showed a statistically significantly higher factor score on F-2 (powerlessness, t=3.852, df=89, p=0.000) than the low-score group. The high-score (>13.7) group on anhedonia-asociality (SANS-4) showed a statistically significantly higher factor score on F-2 (powerlessness, t=2.983, df=89, p=0.004) and P-2 (lifelessness, t=3.272, df=89, p=0.002) than the low-score group.

Insight

The results of the *t*-test of differentiating factor scores between schizophrenic subgroups composed of SAI scores are shown in Table 6. The high-score (>3.29) group on acceptance (SAI-1) showed a statistically significantly lower factor score on F-3 (unusually strong digestive function, t=-2.482, df=89, p=0.015) and higher factor score on P-3 (Fragility, t=2.135, df=89, p=0.036) than the low-score group. The high-score (>1.7) group on hypothetical contradiction (SAI-supplement) showed a statistically significantly lower factor score on F-3 (unusually strong gastrointestinal function, t=-2.348, df=89, p=0.021) than the low-score group.

Other Clinical Characteristics

There was no significant difference between subgroups of body image factor scores in years of hospitalization, age at onset of disease or the daily chlorpromazine-equivalent dose.

Discussion

The factor analysis identified five differentiating factors, which showed that there is body image aberration in schizophrenic patients: dullness in movement, powerlessness, unusually strong digestive function, lifelessness and fragility. These findings, along with those of other investigations (Roehricht and Priebe, 1996; Coleman et al., 1996; Chapman LJ, Chapman and Raulin, 1978), revealed that schizophrenics manifested perceptual and cognitive deficits in body image.

Table 5. Differential BIQ factor scores in high and low score groups of SAPS and SANS. (Study 1)

	Positive symptoms		Negative symptoms	
	SAPS		SANS	
Factors	High	LOW	High	LOW
	SAPS-1		SANS-1	
	Hallucinations		Affective flattening or blunting	
F-1	–	–	–	–
F-2	0.789	0.178*	–	–
F-3	–	–	–	–
P-2	0.608	0.058*	–	–
P-3	–	–	–	–
	SAPS-2		SANS-2	
	Delusions		Alogia	
F-1	–	–	–	–
F-2	0.708	0.208*	–	–
F-3	–	–	–	–
P-2	0.794	-0.033**	–	–
P-3	–	–	–	–
	SAPS-3		SANS-3	
	Bizarre Behaviour		Avolition Apathy	
F-1	–	–	–	–
F-2	–	–	0.805	-0.013**
F-3	–	–	–	–
P-2	–	–	–	–
P-3	–	–	–	–
	SAPS-4		SANS-4	
	Positive formal Thought Disorder		Anhedonia-associality	
F-1	–	–	–	–
F-2	0.723	0.098**	0.718	0.064**
F-3	–	–	–	–

Table 5. (Continued)

	Positive symptoms		Negative symptoms	
P-2	–	–	0.599	-0.082**
P-3	–	–	–	–
	SAPS-5		SANS-5	
	Inappropriate affect		Attention	
F-1	–	–	–	–
F-2	–	–	_	–
F-3	–	–	–	–
	SAPS		SANS	
P-2	–	–	–	–
P-3	–	–	–	–
	SAPS-Total		SANS-Total	
F-1	–	–	–	–
F-2	.729	0.180*	–	–
F-3	–	–	–	–
P-2	0.556	0.067*	–	–
P-3	–	–	–	–

High =High score group. Low=Low score group. *=p<0.05, **=p<0.01.

Table 6. Differential BIQ factor scores in high and low score groups of SAI. (Study 1)

BIQ	SAI		SAI	
Factors	High	Low	High	Low
	SAI-1a.		SAI-1b.	
	Treatment compliance (passive)		Treatment compliance (unprompted)	
F-1	–	–	–	–
F-2	–	–	–	–
F-3	0.047	0.546*	–	–
P-2	–	–	–	–
P-3	0.368	-0.059*	–	–
	SAI-2a.		SAI-2b.	
	Awareness of illness		Awareness of illness	
	(mental, physical)		(mental, psychiatric)	
F-1	–	–	–	–
F-2	–	–	–	–
F-3	–	–	–	–
P-2	–	–	–	
P-3	–	–	–	–
	SAI-2c.			
	Explanation of illness			
F-1	–	–		

Table 6. (Continued)

BIQ	SAI		SAI	
Factors	High	Low	High	Low
F-2	–	–		
F-3	–	–		
P-2	–	–		
P-3	–	–		
	SAI-3a.		SAI-3b.	
	Relabelling		Explanation	
	of psychotic experience		of psychotic experience	
F-1	–	–	–	–
F-2	–	–	–	–
F-3	–	–	–	–
P-2	–	–	–	–
P-3	–	–	–	–
	SAI-total		SAI-supplemental	
			Hypothetical Contradiction	
F-1	–	–	–	–
F-2	–	–	–	–
F-3	–	–	-0.135	0.303*
P-2	–	–	–	–
P-3	–	–	–	–

*=p<0.05.

Among the five differential body image factors, only two factors showed correlation with positive symptoms measured by SAPS: powerlessness and lifelessness, and the same factors correlated with negative symptoms. These results highlighted the close relationships between powerless and lifeless body images and severity in symptoms, both positive and negative, implying that the patients with severe symptoms would have powerless and lifeless body images.

Although the current view is that schizophrenics lack insight (Amador et al. 1994, 1991,; Cuesta and Peralta, 1994), the results of the present study showed that there is variation in degree of insight measured by SAI. The results also showed that acceptance of treatment, as one component of insight, as assessed by the SAI, proved to be related negatively with unusual gastrointestinal function and positively with the fragile body image, showing that patients who comply with treatment have fragile body images and have images of digestive organs that are not too strong. It might be well estimated that the fragile body image and the reduction of strength of images of digestive organs enhance the patients' feeling of needing help, which makes them compliant to treatment. Another insight component that showed a relationship with the deviated body image factor was the double-awareness phase, as assessed by the hypothetical contradiction, a supplemental item of the SAI. This was conceived as the degree of the patient's conviction about the delusion, as it appeared in the recovery from delusion (Sacks et al, 1974), and arising "from rapid oscillations between belief and disbelief." The score suggests "the amenability to test still firmly held beliefs against reality" (Sacks et al, 1974). The degree of double awareness was shown to be inversely related with the image of unusual strength of gastrointestinal function, showing that the patients with flexible amenability to delusional ideas have images of digestive organs that are not very strong.

The overall results proved two out of the five factors that differentiated the schizophrenic from the normal group to be related to positive and negative symptoms and two to insight. It is important that one major differentiating factor, dullness in movement, did not show any correlation with symptoms or insight. During the 1990s, observations focused on the fact that while patients' symptoms were improved markedly by antipsychotic agents, the patients still required assisted living arrangements and could not work in highly competitive situations (Goldberg et al, 1993). The fact that the main part of the body image deviancy assessed by BIQ did not relate to positive or negative symptoms is assumed to have some relation to these observations, and suggests the possibility that the main component of body image deviancy, which is independent from severity of symptoms, is closely related to some deficits that are germane to schizophrenia.

Conclusion

The factor analysis of BIQ showed some aberrant phases of schizophrenics' body image. They were: dullness in movement, powerlessness, unusually strong gastrointestinal function, lifelessness and fragility. Powerlessness and lifelessness proved to be related to positive and negative symptoms and unusually strong gastrointestinal functions and fragility, to insight.

Study 2. Schizophrenics' Body Images: What are They?

Introduction

In Study 1, the attempts with factor analysis to find out the linkage of schizophrenics' aberrant body image with clinical characteristics proved to be exhaustive. However, the results of factor analysis showed that there are some differential body image factors, none of which seemed to relate to an anatomical component of body image of schizophrenia. It was further observed that most of the BIQ differential items were functional and psychological.

Distorted body experiences in schizophrenic patients, especially regarding their images of their body shape or proportions, have been reported since the 1960s. DeLeon et al (1989) denoted dysmorphophobia as a symptom which occurs in a number of different disorders, notably in schizophrenia. Dysmorphophobia as seen in somatoform disorders (1980), body dysmorphic disorder (1987) and delusional disorder, somatic subtype, were included in the Diagnostic and Statistical Manual of Mental Disorders, which produced considerable concern about delusion regarding the appearance of the body. (deLeon et al, 1989; Phillips et al, 1994). There has also been much discussion on distorted body experiences, which are legitimately categorized as psychological derivative imageries, including coenaesthesis (Huber, 1957; Rohricht and Priebe, 1996; Schmoll, 1994). Much concern has been placed on the blurred nature of body boundaries (Quinlan and Harrow, 1974; Fisher S, 1966), and the

Rorschach test has been used to examine the vulnerable characteristics of body boundaries such as penetrability. In spite of all these attempts, clinical relevance of body image aberration remains unclear. It is still uncertain whether or not the body images are deviated in the area of visual imagery, or in feelings about their body such as being hard as stone or being fragile.

Thus, the question of which phase of body image links with symptoms and which to recovery? leads to the next question, "What are schizophrenics' body images, or what are their aberrations?" In this section, attempts were made to clarify this question simply by comparing three hypothetical components of BIQ, that is, anatomical, functional, and psychological, between schizophrenic and non-schizophrenic groups.

Method

Assessment of Body Image Deviation

Body images were assessed using the BIQ. The three BIQ component scores, *anatomical, functional,* and *psychological,* were obtained using scoring system with reverse items. (See, Appendix 1-1.) Items included in each component are shown in the Appendix. (See Appendix 1-3, 1-4 and 1-5.)

Subjects

The study sample consisted of 83 chronic schizophrenics; 44 were men and 39 were women. The mean (SD) age of the patients was 48.2 (10.0) years. All of them were inpatients in chronic psychiatric wards of a mental hospital in Ibaraki Prefecture in Japan. They were diagnosed as schizophrenia, according to DSM-IV criteria (Subtypes: 20 Paranoid types, 36 Disorganized types, 23 Residual types, 4 Undifferentiated types). The mean (SD) duration of hospitalization was 23.7 (10.5) years, and the mean (SD) age of onset was 24.2 (7.0) years old. Their mean (SD) dose of neuroleptics was 437.0 (396.9) mg/day of chrolpromazine equivalent dose. The group with anxiety disorders was comprised of 43 patients with anxiety disorders in DSM-IV, including 23 men and 20 women. They were outpatients of a private clinic in Ibaraki Prefecture in Japan. The mean (SD) age was 39.1 (14.1) years old. The normal control group of study 1 was used. All of the study participants were informed of the purpose of the study and actively participated with a written informed consent. (See Table 7.)

Table 7. Demographic and clinical characteristics of subjects. (Study 2)

	Schizophrenia	Anxiety Disorders	Normals
	(N=83)	(N=43)	N=177
Demographic characteristics			
Mean Age	48.2	39.1	44.9
Gender (Male %)	53.0	53.4	44.0
Clinical characteristics of the schizophrenic patients			
	Mean (Range)		
Age of Onset	24.2 (14-45)		

Table 7. (Continued)

	Schizophrenia	Anxiety Disorders	Normals
	(N=83)	(N=43)	N=177
Years of Hospitalization	23.7 (3-47)		
Dose of CPZ (mg/day)	437.0 (30-1256)		

Data Analysis

Means of the three BIQ component scores were compared among groups with schizophrenia, anxiety disorders and normals using ANOVA, followed by multiple comparisons using the Tukey method. The means of each item score of the differential component scores obtained were compared between the schizophrenic and non-schizophrenic groups using ANOVA.

Results

The results of ANOVA are shown in Table 8, and the results of succeeded multiple comparisons are shown in Table 12. Statistically significant group differences in means were found in the BIQ functional component score (F=12.478, df=2/284, p=0.000). Further multiple comparisons of differences of means showed a statistically significant difference between groups with schizophrenia and anxiety disorders (p =0.021), and between groups with schizophrenia and normal groups (p = 0.000). There was no statistically significant difference among the three diagnostic groups in the BIQ anatomical component score or in the BIQ psychological component score.

The mean scores of BIQ functional items, which composed the differential component, were further compared between schizophrenic and non-schizophrenic groups. Eight out of 17 items showed statistically significant differences, including being weak (F=7.262, df=2, p<.001), being liable to get sick (F=10.810, df=2, p<.000), moving slowly (F=6.065, df=2, p<.003), being poor at athletics (F=7.743, df=2, p<.001),, being liable to lose balance(F=5.092, df=2, p<.007), walking slowly(F=3.314, df=2, p<.038), being unable to work in dark rooms(F=10.415, df=2, p<.000), and having weak teeth (F=5.614, df=2, p<.004). The means of each functional item are shown in Table 9.

Table 8. Group means of BIQ component Scores. (Study 2)

	Schizophrenia	Anxiety Disorders	Normals	
	(N=83)	(N=43)	(N=177)	F
Anatomical	80.6	70.71	79.1	1.818
Functional	78.4	73.07	71.4	12.478***
Psychological	78.4	84.77	72.5	2.800
Total	238.8	228.34	223.1	18.046***

*P<0.05, **P<0.01, ***P<0.001.

Table 9. Means of BIQ-Functional items of three diagnostic groups. (Study 2)

	SC	AD	NO	F
01. My body is weak.	3.853	3.558	3.175	7.264***
03. I often get sick.	3.734	3.558	2.945	10.810***
09. I move slowly.	4.253	3.857	3.649	6.065**
13. I am good at athletics.®	4.465	4.432	3.626	7.743**
17. I often lose my balance.	3.790	3.566	3.153	5.092**
21. I walk slowly.	4.409	3.690	4.101	3.314*
37. I can work well in dark rooms. ®	3.570	3.418	2.783	10.415***
47. My teeth are weak.	4.817	4.209	4.079	5.614**

®=reverse item.
*P<0.05, **P<0.01, ***P<0.001.

Discussion

Results of this study showed aberration restricted to functional imageries, revealing that there are both intact and deficient phases in schizophrenics' body images. Of three hypothesized components, that is, anatomical, functional, and psychological body images, only functional imageries proved to be deviant.

The results of the comparisons of means of the various functional items between groups showed that differences included three categories of ill-functional body imageries. First was vulnerability to illness, including images of being weak and of being liable to get sick. Second was difficulty in manipulating their bodies, including images of being unable to work in dark rooms, being poor at athletics, walking slowly and of moving slowly. The third category was unusual concern over gastrointestinal functions reflected in having weak teeth.

Conclusion

Via the analysis of three hypothetical components of BIQ, the schizophrenic body image deviation proved to be comprised of deviation in functional imageries.

Study 3. Depression and Body Imagein Chronic Schizophrenia

Introduction

Although mood disorders are conventionally viewed as nosologically distinct from schizophrenia, depression in schizophrenia has been recognized from the time of Mayer-Gross (1920) and Bleuler (1911/1950). Comorbid depressive signs and symptoms (DSS) in schizophrenia were earlier described as postpsychotic depression (McGlaschan and

Carpenter, 1976), resulting from realization of disability once psychosis has abated and insight is recovered. A second view is described as post-treatment depression in which neuroleptic medication causes depression in schizophrenia (Van Puttan and May, 1978 ;Galdi, 1983). The concept has been further elaborated by Van Putten and May (1978), who argued that depression in schizophrenia might be specifically associated with extrapyramidal side effects of neuroleptic medication. A third view relates depression to the schizophrenic process itself. According to this hypothesis, depression forms an integral part of the illness, predicting that depressive symptoms would be most prevalent during the acute phase of illness and subside with treatment (Knights and Hirsch, 1981; Hirsch, 1982).

Recently, DSS have become a target of treatment because novel antipsychotic agents introduce new avenues that may differentially affect schizophrenic signs and symptoms, including depression (Pickar, 1995; Tollefson et al., 1998), and its association with a higher risk of suicide and self-harm (Siris, 1991; Hu et al., 1991; Drake and Cotton, 1986; Caldwell and Gottesman, 1990; Cohen et al., 1990; Roy et al., 1983) has been highlighted. There are studies that reported depressive schizophrenics attempt at unusual self-mutilation (Feldman, 1988; Burgess, 1991; Martin and Gattaz, 1991; Weiser et al., 1993; Kennedy and Feldmann, 1994), which suggest a close relationship between DSS in schizophrenia to body image aberrations.

The report in this section looks at depression in schizophrenia by detecting its unique relationship to patients' body image using BIQ.

Method

Subjects

The subjects in study 1 were used. (See Table 1.)

Assessment of Depression

Depression was assessed by Zung's Self-rating Depression Scale (SDS, Zung, 1965). The SDS scores ranged from 24 to 64, and their mean (SD) was 40.0 (7.9). Based on the distribution, the (schizophrenic and normal) depressive groups were comprised of those who scored 48 or higher, which included 20.3% of all subjects, including schizophrenicc and normal populations. The non-depressive groups were comprised of those who scored 32 or lower, which included 18.9% of all subjects.

Data Analysis

The means of the factor scores obtained in study 1 were compared between the depressive (SDS scores >=48) and non-depressive (SDS scores =<32) groups in schizophrenic and normal control samples, respectively, using *t*-tests. In addition, 59 item scores of BIQ were compared between high and low score groups in these comparative sets using *t*-tests.

Results

Based on the results of the *t*-test of means of obtained factor scores of schizophrenic depressive and non-depressive groups, 5 of these proved to be factors that differentiated the two groups. These factors and their interpretations are factor A-3 (roundness, t=-2.420, df=37, *p*=0.021), factor F-2 (powerlessness, t=2.407, df=38, *p*=0.021), factor F-3(Unusually strong gastrointestinal function, t=-2.588, df=38, *p*=0.014), factor P-1 (Dissatisfuction, t=2.491, df=38, *p*=0.015) and factor P-2 (Lifelessness, t=2.556, df=38, *p*=0.015). Among these factors, significant differences were found among normal population in factor P-1 (t= 5.010, df=40, p=0.000), and factor P-2 (t=2.756, df=40, *p*=0.009), showing that schizophrenic and normal groups had common relationships of depression to body image along with these factors. The other three of the five factors did not differentiate depressive and non-depressive groups in normal samples. Also, there was no factor differentiating depressive and non-depressive group uniquely found in the normal samples. (See Table 10.)

Table 10. BIQ Factors differentiating depressive and non-depressive state. (Study 3)

Factors	Schizophrenic		Control	
	D	Non-D	D	Non-D
A-1	_	_	_	_
A-2	_	_	_	_
A-3	-2.220	.449*	_	_
F-1	_	_	_	_
F-2	.794	-.030*	_	_
F-3	-.165	.620*	_	_
P-1	.262	-.513*	.764	-.331***
P-2	.751	-.198*	.411	-.356*
P-3	_	_	_	_

D=Depressive group, Non-D=Non-depressive group. *P<.0.05, **P<0.01, ***P<0.001.

There were BIQ items which differentiated depressive and non-depressive groups only in schizophrenic samples. These were; having small eyes, being not meager, being weak, being clumsy with hands, having unusually strong stomach, having strong heart, having strong bowels, being underdeveloped, feeling cold, being dissatisfied, not minding being touched by others, and being getting worse. Schizophrenic and normal control samples shared the most of the differentiating items in the psychological element. (See table 11.)

Table 11. BIQ items differentiating depressive and non-depressive state. (Study 3)

	Schizophrenics		Normals	
BIQ items	D	Non-D	D	Non-D
Anatomical				
18. I have small eyes.	4.200	3.181*		
44. My body is not meager.®	4.266	3.000**		
Functional				

Table 11. (Continued)

	Schizophrenics		Normals	
BIQ items	D	Non-D	D	Non-D
01. My body is weak.	4.600	3.454*		
03. I often get sick.	4.400	3.000*	3.461	2.655*
17. I often lose my balance.			4.461	2.714***
25. I am clumsy with my hands.	4.833	3.181**		
37. I can work well in dark rooms. ®	5.666	4.181**	3.692	4.655*
38. My stomach is not unusually strong. ®	3.600	5.181**		
42. My heart is strong. ®	3.933	2.272**		
53. My bowels are unusually strong.	3.766	5.000*		
Psychological				
06. My body is underdeveloped.	.3.866	2.636*		
07. My body is clean.®			3.153	2.413**
10. My body is defective.	4.400	3.363*	4.692	3.448**
11. My body feels cold.	4.233	5.363*		
12. My body is beautiful.®	4.333	3.272*	4.769	3.482***
22. I seldom feel tired.®			5.461	4.206**
23. My mood is numb.	3.833	5.090*	2.000	4.724***
27. I am satisfied with my body. ®	3.200	4.727*		
31. I am always cheerful. ®			3.923	2.931**
32. My body is unattractive.			5.153	3.931***
34. I always feel sick.	4.433	3.181*	4.615	3.413***
43. I don't mind being touched by others. ®	4.866	3.636*		
45. I seldom get excited			2.833	4.275**
46. My health is getting better. ®	5.000	3.900*		
49. I am seldom tense.	2.400	3.909**	2.076	3.241**
59. I always feel energetic.®	4.666	3.363**	4.307	3.137**

D=Depressive group, Non-D=Non-depressive group. *P<.0.05, **P<0.01, ***P<0.001.

Discussion

The depression assessed by SDS correlated to 5 factors of body image assessed by BIQ. The findings further demonstrated that 3 among these 5 factors correlated with depression in schizophrenic groups, interpreted as roundness, dullness in movement, and unusually strong gastrointestinal function, none of which differentiated depressive from non-depressive group in normal subjects. It would be reasonable to assume that there is some close link between depression and body image, which is unique and specific to schizophrenia.

Dissatisfied and lifeless body images were found to be related to depression in schizophrenic as well as in normal samples. Dissatisfaction and lifelessness would be a common body image factors they shared regardless of diagnosis. In the schizophrenic sample, three differentiating factors were further observed, one anatomical factor, and two functional factors. It was observed that the more the schizophrenic patients becomes depressed, the less round and the less powerful their imagined body becomes and that the more they depressed, the less powerful their gastrointestinal function becomes in their body images. The results of the comparisons of means of each BIQ item also demonstrated that the variety of functional body image items differentiated depressive from non-depressive patients in the schizophrenic sample. The concern on bodily function proved to be prominent in schizophrenic depressive patients.

These observations may suggest that these depression-related body images in schizophrenia have characteristics, which lead to the anticipation of the serious corporeal deterioration of becoming immovable. This close linkage between depression and undesirable functional body images in schizophrenic patients would be connected with the self-mutilation or higher risk of self-harm observed in schizophrenia.

Part III. Studies Using Rorschach Test: Subsidiary Findings

Study 4. A Unique Rorschach Response Observed in Schizophrenic Patients

Introduction

Although recognized as closely linked with psychopathology, distortion of body image has seldom been studied in schizophrenia. The major cause of the neglect of this concept is methodological, i.e., the difficulty in developing assessment techniques. In this section, a new finding concerning body image of schizophrenia, as observed in their Rorschach responses, is reported.

In the attempts to detect body image aberration in the studies using the BIQ, we found that responses that evoke images of a mass of flesh are often seen in schizophrenic Rorschach responses. This was first noticed in the response of a schizophrenic patient (Case A of this study) as "This looks like a mass of flesh of some kind of animal, though I cannot specify which," to Card VI. This response followed to the failure to construct the response "a gorilla" in Card IV, in which she could not identify its legs, arms, or head. According to this Rorschach sequence, a process is assumed to exist in schizophrenic thought that the their bodies are becoming a mere mass of flesh, as if they were being vivisected though still alive, which forms a core of fear of schizophrenic patients. Difficulty in identifying legs, arms, and head of perceived animals or human beings also proved to be a process of perceiving "a mass of flesh."

Starting with these observations, an attempt was made to explore similar responses in schizophrenics' Rorschach responses, and it was found that these responses are quite common in schizophrenic patients. We call the characteristics revealed in these responses as body image "becoming a mass of flesh" and present the hypothesis that this might form a core characteristic of body image of schizophrenia.

Responses such as "mass of flesh", or "muscles in the shoulder of a man," are typical mass of flesh responses because the image of a mass of flesh is clearly verbalized in these responses. Responses such as "a rat without legs" or "a girl, but I cannot see her hands" are also mass-of-flesh responses, because these responses, though indirect, vaguely imagine a mass of flesh through the diminution of head, legs, and arms and emphasis on the trunk.

Four cases are presented. All of them were inpatients of a chronic care ward of a mental hospital in Ibaraki Prefecture and were diagnosed as schizophrenia according to DSM-IV. All patients were informed of the purpose of the study and actively participated with written informed consent. The socio-demographic and clinical characteristics, such as illness type, onset age, years of hospitalization, BPRS scores (Overall and Gorham, 1962), and daily dose of neuroleptics, are shown in Table 12.

Table 12. Demographic and clinical characteristics of subjects. (Study 4)

	Case A	Case B	Case C	Case D
Age	62	46	33	28
Gender	Female	Female	Male	Female
Years of education	9	7	13	12
Years of employment	2	0	0	4
Illnessl types	Paranoid	Disorganized	Disorganized	Residual
Age at onset	19	16	19	22
Years of hospitalization	37	30	33	5
BPRS	51	49	64	25
Daily dose of neuroleptics (mg)	400	1525	175	350

Case Reports

Case A

Miss A was a 62-year-old woman. She was born to a farmer in Ibaraki Prefecture in Japan as the first of seven children. After she graduated from high school, she went to Tokyo and worked as a housekeeper, but one year later she became restless, sleepless, and went back home. At the age of 22, she was admitted to the hospital with prominent delusional experiences. She left the hospital once, but soon left home, wandered around, stole food from a store and was returned the hospital. Since then, she has been in the hospital for 37 years.

In a semi-structured interview, she said, "A fox is controlling me. He exchanges my body with that of a victim of a traffic accident, so that I feel great pain in my legs, head, and arms. The fox is one of the foxes I keep at home. He changes my body because he gets money through traffic accidents. I am a splendid and super woman. If I had not been ill, I would have made a country. I sculpted on the moon as well as the sun."

In the Rorschach Test, she gave one response per card and gave in seven responses among ten animals with unclear or absent legs, arms, or head, or irregular emphasis on the legs. "Two elephants, but the legs are too short for elephants"(Card II). "A bat, legs are just like those of a bat" (Card V). "An animal I have never seen before. It looks like a gorilla, but this has no head, no legs, and no arms" (Card IV, IX). "A shrimp, with big tails and many small legs"(Card IX).

Case B

Miss B was a 46-year-old woman. She was a third of four children in the family of a public official. She suffered from tuberculosis in the junior high school. One day she was made a fun of by her classmates and refused to go to school. At the age of sixteen, she began to speak in monologues and to spend almost all day in bed. She showed delusions and hallucinations, and entered into the hospital when she was seventeen years old.

In the interview, she said, "I have been suffering from hallucinations everyday for twenty or thirty years. I hear the voice of a middle-aged woman, and she always says bad things about me. It causes severe pain in my shoulder. But I still continue knitting. When I brush my teeth, I feel like I am dying. When I am in bed, and also I am walking, germs move and frighten me, and dogs and cats are lying on me. All animals are transparent so that I cannot see them but they certainly exist."

She presented feelings of "being pressed" in 3 responses among a total of 7. "A calf oppressed by a fixed butterfly" (Card II). "Human beings are pressed down with their hands on the floor" (Card III). "A crab which is compressed, narrow in width" (Card X). She also showed an image of becoming a mass in the response, "A rat, there are no legs" to Card VIII.

Case C

Mr. C was a 55-year-old man. He was born the fourth child of a wealthy family in Tokyo. His father owned a company, and he went to private school. When he was in university, in the first year, he went to a supermarket with the group of his friends to steal some small things. He was expelled from the university. Since then, he complained of anxiety at meeting people, and visited many clinics for medication and psychotherapy, but he gradually came to stay at home almost all day. When he was 22 years old, he entered the hospital with prominent delusions and hallucinations.

In the interview, the patient said, "I suffer from nightmares every night. It is a dream of hell and I feel I cannot survive any more with these ominous ideas. I cannot concentrate. I am slow in thinking. And I have become old-fashioned. Somebody is talking ill of me. I feel suspected as a criminal every time a crime is broadcast on the television. It is because I know the names of the criminals, so that this is my referential delusion."

He showed five human movement responses, none of which identified the agent. "Hitting each other with both hands" (Card I), "Washing" (Card III), "Dancing" (Card VI), "Being astonished (Card VII), and "Talking, with each other" (Card X). He also showed over-clarification of ages in his human percepts, as "old" (Card II), "middle-aged" (Cards III, X), and "young" (Card VII). These estimations of age without evidence suggest the possibility that there might be strong conflict in his subjective inability to experience time, from which he feels excluded.

Case D

Miss D is a 28-year-old woman. She was the second of two children of a family of an artisan in Ibaraki Prefecture. When she was 16 years old, she felt that her classmates are talking ill of her so she refused to go to school. She once consulted with a psychologist. After she graduated from high school, she went to Tokyo and worked for a large company there for five years. When her mother got sick, she came back home to see her mother. Soon after her mother died, she became sleepless, violent especially toward her father, suffered from hallucinations and entered the hospital at the age of 23. After her admission, the hallucinations disappeared, and she returned home to stay several times, although she was not successful in staying home every time because of her violent behaviour toward her father.

In the interview, she said, "I feel miserable because I am under the protection of my father who is so slovenly that he spends a lot of money on bicycle races. My father hit me. But it is because I poured water on him. I am worried that I cannot be independent, though I am old enough to be. To tell the truth, I want to be a child of my elder sister."

She presented the body image as a mass of flesh in the response, "A crab, with torso with a carapace and nippers" (Card III), in which the mass-of-flesh image was covered with the hard shield of a crab and the impression of the whole response was aggressive and defensive, ready for fight. She also showed withdrawal of the body from the outer world in the response, "A piece of clothing, too showy for me." She showed helpless feelings in the response, "A flower, with leaves hanging down and connected with the roots in this way" (Card IX). In this response, the psychological process is presented as a feeling of helplessness that was developed into an attempt to confirm that she was related to her support system.

Discussion

The body image becoming a mass of flesh was seen in four cases as a common characteristics of body image, regardless of their variety of illness type, of degree of severity of symptoms assessed by BPRS, life history and daily dose of neuroleptic medication. Clarification of how this mass-of-flesh image is expressed and is related to the patients' clinical pictures is necessary. Three questions need to be discussed with regard to these patients: (1) Is mass-of-flesh image really related to delusion?: (2) Is it related to hallucinatory behaviour? (3) Is it related to symptoms other than delusional and hallucinatory experiences?

Case A refers to the first question. In this case, body image as a mass of flesh was expressed in a typical form as "a mass of flesh of some animal with a bamboo stick." From this response, it is assumed that she has a catastrophic fear of her body being exposed to the outer world without protection, being penetrated. It is further guessed that this fear is elaborated into a delusional belief to clarify and explain its origin, by thinking that a naughty fox exchanged her body with that of a victim of a traffic accident, and that the fox is one of many foxes she kept at home.

Case B exemplifies to the second question. In this case, the body image of becoming a mass of flesh was expressed as "a rat without arms and legs" and also as "a crab which was compressed" and "a calf that was oppressed by a butterfly." These responses imply that body image as becoming a mass of flesh modified into more sensory form as "being pressed" and developed into a hallucination. She suffered from being oppressed at shoulder presumably caused by a middle-aged woman's voice. She also suffered from being oppressed by germs creeping on her and by transparent animals lying on her.

Case C refers to the third question. In this case, the agents in human Rorschach percepts are frequently not identified. Omission of the head is an indirect expression of body image as a mass of flesh. The lack of identification of the agents of the human percepts implies his avoidance of committing himself to the percepts. With this withdrawal, he tries to maintain distance by regarding the whole situation in which he lives as if it were a fiction, acted on a stage, and regarding himself as an audience. He described his own symptoms as "referential delusion" as if others observe him and felt himself "like a criminal who appears on television". His over-concern about age and many attempts to guess age without enough evidence would be derived phenomenon from this withdrawal from the real world, in which time passes, into a fictional narcissistic world, in which there is no lapse of time. He is worried about "becoming old-fashioned." This concern toward age seems consistent with the age-disorientation of schizophrenia (Crow and Johnstone, 1980; Crow and Stevens, 1978). It was reported that 25% of the schizophrenic patients mistake their own ages by more than 5 years.

In Case D, the mass-of-flesh percepts appeared in the perception, "A crab, with a torso with a carapace and nippers" (Card III). A mass of flesh was seen in the elimination of the legs with armor. This is consistent with her clinical picture, in which her violent acting-out is a prominent problem. As the risk of violence has come to be one of the current issues of schizophrenia (Taylor, 1995; Fottrell,1980; Humphreys et al., 1992) the present finding seems to relate to some illness-specific risk factor to evoke violence in schizophrenic patients. In this case, it is assumed that an "armored mass-of-flesh body image" would be a compromised product of an aggressive premorbid personality and schizophrenic illness.

The body image as becoming a mass of flesh is considered to have four connotations. First, it suggests an image of the body, which is still alive, though exposed to the outer world. Second, it suggests an image of the body that is helplessly threatened and unprotected. Third, it suggests an image of the body that is unmovable. Fourth, it suggests an image of the body that is weakened and helpless. These would constitute an image of potential catastrophe concerning the patients' own body.

The image of becoming a mass of flesh was recognized in two stages. Stage 1 is presented directly with reference to "a mass of muscles" or "mass of flesh," as seen as a typical response one. Stage 2 as presented indirectly as an animal or a human being without legs or arms, or without clarifying them, in which the mass of flesh is vaguely imagined through the diminution of head or legs. In observation of these four cases above, stage 1 presumably works with delusion, especially being closely linked with bizarre delusions and enhancing psychological factors for it. Stage 2 would exist as a rather general, though underlying, disposition in schizophrenic patients. In the case of stage 2, it was further shown that image of becoming a mass of flesh leads to some readiness for age-disorientation as one of the major thought disorders, as well as violent acting-out behaviours, so that one of the future topics to be discussed should be the effect of the image of becoming a mass of flesh on the formation of a variety of schizophrenic symptoms.

Conclusion

Rorschach responses that imply the body images of becoming a mass of flesh were shown in four chronic schizophrenic cases. The body images of becoming a mass of flesh were experienced in two forms: one is experienced by the percept of a mass of muscles. The other is by percepts of an animal or a human being with diminished legs, head, or arms. In studying four cases carefully, these responses were found regardless of the illness type, duration of illness, life history, and neuroleptic doses, but they related not only to delusional and hallucinatory symptoms but also to some other thought disorders such as age-disorientation as well as violence. Because this is just an initial phase of the study, further studies are required to determine whether this finding is a general intrinsic trend of schizophrenia or not.

Study 5. A mass of flesh: schizophrenic Rorschach percepts

Introduction

The Rorschach test is important in the diagnosis of schizophrenia. Since 1966, 1728 studies using the Rorschach test, among which 126 were concerned with the diagnosis of schizophrenia, have been indexed in Medline. Rorschach protocols have been documented in thought disorders, sometimes in terms of ego impairment, to provide information concerning diagnosis of schizophrenia. Rappaport et al. (1968) are historically credited with systematically identifying deviant aspects of the patient's verbal responses to the inkblot. Attempts have been made to develop specific criteria on the Rorschach designed to make a more accurate assessment of thought disorders, including the Delta Index (Watkins and Stauffacher, 1952), Thought Disorder Index (Johnston and Holzman, 1979), and Schizophrenia Index (Exner, 1974, 1978, 1986a, 1986b, 1991, 1993; Mason et al., 1985). Earlier, methods were developed to assess "primary process" manifestations (Holt, 1977; Meloy, 1984) or boundary disturbance manifestations (Quinlan and Harrow, 1974). During the 1970s to 1980s, methods to assess object relations were developed to differentiate borderline personality disorders from schizophrenia (Urist, 1977; Kwawer, 1980). In the 1990s, Wagner and Frye (Wagner and Frye, 1990) reported the diagnostic implication of the "fragmented" Rorschach W:D (Whole Responses vs. Detail Responses) ratio in schizophrenia, and Perry developed perseveration measures (Perry and Braff, 1998). One of the most widely used of these Rorschach criteria for the evaluation of schizophrenia is the Comprehensive System's Schizophrenia Indices, SCZI (Exner, 1974; Mason et al., 1985). The Comprehensive System began to pay more attention to the importance of systematically measuring unusual verbalizations and identifying reliable test signs that capture a range of aberrations in thought and language. The diagnostic indicators of disordered thinking in Exner's approach pointed to large differences between schizophrenia and control subjects, confirming an impairment of perceptual accuracy, reality testing and reduced emotional control (Di-Nuovo et al., 1988), and the Exner Rorschach was judged to be a valid test for schizophrenia (Vincent and Harman, 1991; Hilsenroth et al., 1998). Another index, the Ego Impairment Index, proved to differentiate among schizophrenics according to the severity of their ego impairment (Perry et al., 1992). Recently, investigators have placed much emphasis on Rorschach indications for thought disorders in regard to sensorimotor gating abnormalities or other information processing in the neurocognitive context (Perry and Braff, 1994; Perry et al., 1999).

In the previous section (study 4), a new finding was reported concerning Rorschach percepts of schizophrenia, that images of a mass of flesh were often seen in schizophrenic Rorschach responses. This was first noticed in the Rorschach response to Card VI of a middle-aged female (Case A) with chronic schizophrenia in the statement, "This looks like a mass of flesh of some kind of animal, although I cannot specify which animal." Before producing this response, the patient had failed to make the response of " a gorilla" to Card IV, in which she could not identify its arms, legs or head. According to these Rorschach sequences, it would be considered that if the patient has failed to see the legs and arms, a gorilla is perceived as a mass of flesh. A similar response was found in another middle-aged male with chronic schizophrenia, who responded to Card IX, "Part of a naked man, the swelling muscles of his shoulder." This patient also responded to Card VIII, "The carcass of an animal. Only bones here, for the flesh is gone." In this response, he imagined a mass of flesh and quickly eliminated it by thinking of it as having been taken away in his fantasy. The third patient, a middle-aged female with chronic schizophrenia, who gave another such response, by responding to Card VIII, saying "Two seals. They are seals, because their legs and arms are quite short. They look like muscles. Only the muscles of seals. With backbones here." In this response, she saw two aquatic animals that have intrinsically diminished (short) legs and arms, and this image soon became muscles with backbones.

Starting with these findings, the attempts were made further to find similar responses in their Rorschach percepts. It was found that the responses in which a mass of flesh or muscles are explicitly verbalized are not often seen in their Rorschach percepts, but that the responses with the same implications in modified and implicit forms, especially in the form of animals or human beings with diminution of head, legs or arms, were quite common in schizophrenic patients.

Although apparently different, these responses share the common characteristic of revealing the perception of a mass of flesh in the Rorschach pattern. The author called the above percept "a mass of flesh" (MF) and considered that the implications of the MFs should be studied further in the diagnosis of schizophrenia. In order to detect MFs reliably, inclusion and exclusion criteria for MFs were developed which describes the details to identify the MFs.

First, this study is an attempt to develop inclusion criteria for detecting these responses based on these observations. Second, to examine whether perception of MFs is characteristic in schizophrenia or not, the presence or absence of the MFs was examined in the Rorschach protocols of patients in the diagnostic groups of acute schizophrenia, anxiety disorders according to DSM-IV criteria, and healthy adults.

Method

Inclusion and Exclusion Criteria for the MF Percept

The idea that schizophrenics produce percepts of a mass of flesh evolved through our earlier observations in the evaluation of 7 chronic schizophrenia patients. Thereafter, particular attention was given to the responses of 69 consecutive chronic schizophrenic patients (76 in total) to confirm whether or not they produced any response which had a connotation of a mass of flesh or its implicit representation, mainly reflected in diminution of head, arms or legs, of any living thing. After it was confirmed that 75 out of 76 (98%) chronic schizophrenic patients produced some MFs, a list of criteria for MFs was made to detect them reliably.

MFs are, in their explicit and typical form, responses in which a mass of flesh or muscle is explicitly verbalized. The MFs, in their implicit forms, include responses in which diminution of arm, leg, and head is mentioned. In these responses, absence, unusual shortness or vagueness of arms, legs or head is verbalized. The things or living things with a mass-like shape, or perceived as folded or unfolded, are also included because these responses reflect the image of a mass of flesh or the process of becoming a mass of flesh or its denial. Exclusion criteria were made as a guide to exclude misleading responses. Inclusion and exclusion criteria are summarized in Appendix 2.

Test Administration and Scoring

All Rorschach tests were administered by the present authors. The presence or absence of any response that fit the criteria was examined in each case. The cases were divided into two groups, that is, one with MFs and one without.

Inter-Rater Reliability

Inter-rater agreement was determined by evaluating the MFs according to the protocols of 20 chronic schizophrenics. Independent ratings was made by two raters. Nineteen among 20 protocols were scored as showing MF (MF +) by two independent scorers, and 95% inter-rater agreement was obtained.

Subjects

The socio-demographic data of the subjects used for evaluation of the MFs are shown in Table 13. The chronic schizophrenic patients were those of Study 2, who agreed to participate to the study using the Rorschach test. There were 41 men and 35 women. The mean (SD) age of the patients was 49.4 (9.4) years. The mean (SD) chlorpromazine-equivalent dose was 474.8 (406.3) mg. Twenty-two acute schizophrenic patients, 10 male and 12 female, are inpatients of a hospital in a Tokyo suburb. The Rorschach test was administered within one month after their first admission. Their mean (SD) age was 21.8 (3.3) years. All of them were medicated, and the mean (SD) chlorpromazine-equivalent dose was 1082.3 (536.8) mg. All of them had been diagnosed with schizophrenia, according to DSM-IV criteria. Thirty patients with anxiety disorders according to DSM-IV, 16 male and 14 female, were outpatients of a private clinic in Tokyo. Their mean (SD) age was 35.9 (13.4) years. Twenty-eight healthy adults, 14 men and 14 women, were graduate students, hospital staff members, businessmen, office employees, and housewives. The mean (SD) age was 34.1 (12.8) years old. All normal adults were demonstrated to be healthy by administering General Health Questionnaire (Goldberg, 1972; Goldberg and Williams, 1988). Written informed consent was also obtained. (See Table 13.)

Table 13. Demographic characteristics of subjects. (Study 5.)

	Schizophrenia		Anxiety Disorders	Nprmals
	Chronic	Acute		
	(N=76)	(N=22)	(N=30)	(N=22)
Mean Age	49.4	21.8	35.9	34.1
Gender (% male)	53.9	45.5	53.3	50.0

Statistics

The number of subjects perceiving MFs and those not perceiving MF was calculated in each diagnostic group.

Results

Seventy-five out of 76 chronic schizophrenic patients (98%) saw MFs. All 22 acute schizophrenic patients saw MFs. Twenty-eight out of 30 patients with anxiety disorders did not perceive MF. None of the healthy adults saw the MF. It would be reasonable to regard the MFs as characteristic of schizophrenia. The number of subjects perceiving MFs (MF+) and those not perceiving MF (MF-) in schizophrenic and non-schizophrenic groups are shown in Table 14 ($x^2 = 11.308$, df=1, p=0.001).

Both of two patients with anxiety disorders who perceived MFs were young adolescent males and had brief psychotic episodes in their life histories. One patient with chronic schizophrenia who did not perceive MF was a middle-aged male patient who scored the least total response to the inkblots. (His total response was less than ten.)

Table 14. MFs in schizophrenic and non-schizophrenic groups. (Study 5)

	Schizophrenic		Non-schizophrenic	
	Acute	Chronic	Anxiety Disorders	Normal
	(N=22)	(N=76)	(N=30)	(N=28)
MF+	22	75	2	0
MF-	0	1	28	28

Discussion

The primary contribution of this investigation is to find that Rorschach percepts of a mass of flesh are characteristic of schizophrenia. It was found that although there are some differences in their responses, the perception of a mass of flesh in Rorschach inkblot stimuli was broadly seen as living things with diminished arms, legs or head. By developing inclusion and exclusion criteria for MFs, detection of MFs would become easier and more reliable. To test whether the perception of MFs in inkblots is unique to schizophrenia or not, we examined the Rorschach Test data of 22 acute schizophrenia, 30 anxiety disorders and 28 healthy adults. Ninety-seven out of 98 schizophrenic patients saw MFs, although only two out of 30 patients with anxiety disorders saw MFs. Further, healthy adults did not see any MF. Thus, MFs proved to be characteristic of schizophrenia.

An index for detecting such responses is particularly important because it provides a tool for detecting schizophrenia in its early phase. Ninety-eight percent of chronic schizophrenics, as well as 100% of acute schizophrenic patients, perceived MFs. The perception of MFs might exist from the time of onset and therefore be able to detect a very early phase of schizophrenia, suggesting the diagnostic predictive value of MF perception. As a greater understanding of the nature of schizophrenia has refocused attention on the early course of psychosis in the from of early detection and intervention around the onset (McGlashan and Johannessen, 1996) the inclusion and exclusion criteria would have more value if MFs are found in the prodrome of schizophrenia.

The findings that schizophrenic patients produce MF percepts may lead to improvement of our understanding of thought disorder of schizophrenia. The use of the Rorschach test in the study of thought disorder is well established. However, using the Rorschach test for the purpose of eliciting perceptual deficits, manifested in global and affective percepts such as MFs, might provide a new opportunity to understand the cognitive dysfunction of schizophrenia patients.

Conclusion

The Rorschach test was given to schizophrenic and non-schizophrenic subjects to determine whether schizophrenic patients more frequently produced the "mass of flesh" percept than the non-schizophrenic groups did.

Part IV. Discussion and Conclusion

Discussion

The major findings of the studies on schizophrenics' body image aberration in this chapter are: (1) There is some aberration in schizophrenics' body image. (2) There are aberrant as well as intact phases in their body images. (3) Aberration was found in functional imageries, while anatomical imageries are intact. (4) Aberration is independent of symptoms and conventional neuroleptic medication.

The main questions raised in the introduction were whether aberration comes from symptoms or is an effect of neuroleptics, and whether it is remediable or not. What the components of body image are and which phase of body image is aberrant in schizophrenia was the first question we tried to answer by attempts at classification of body image items by factor analysis. Nine body image factors were obtained, and some factors proved to differentiate schizophrenics from normal controls. Although these factors were variously named, after rather exhaustive attempts, the only discrete common feature among factor-analytic studies was that functional imageries may contribute substantially to the factors that meaningfully differentiated groups or were related to depression. In addition, almost no significant correlation was found between aberrant body image factors and clinical characteristics such as symptoms, insight, or neuroleptic dosage. The results of Study 1 showed that when each component of symptoms and insight was cross-validated to the BIQ factors, there were some symptoms and some insight components related to body image factors; however, the overall results showed their relationship was quite weak. The only strong evidence gained through these studies was the fact that there are some differential body image factors, most of which seemed to relate to functional body imageries, but none of which seemed to relate to the anatomical component of body image of schizophrenia.

Thus the question of which phase of body image links with symptoms and which to recovery? leads to the next question, "What are the body images of schizophrenics and what is aberrant for them?" In Study 2, attempts were made to clarify this question simply by comparing three hypothetical components of body image, that is, anatomical, functional, and psychological, between schizophrenic and non-schizophrenic groups. The results showed clearly that anatomical, that is, the visual or the spatial, component is intact in schizophrenia and limited their aberration mainly to functional component.

The fact that schizophrenics have aberrant body images in function, i.e., they have unmovable body images, is controversial with regard to the possibility that it reflects perseverance in motor activity. Schizophrenic patients might have difficulty in the shifting the response set in motor activity in light of the feedback that a previous response was incorrect and consequently "persevere" in making the same response, creating difficulty in movement cognition. Perseveration is a cardinal feature of frontal lobe disease (Bilder and Goldberg, 1987). It is one of the presenting basic neurocognitive deficits, observed since the time of Bleuler (1911/1950), who wrote that schizophrenic patients "remain fixed to the same circle of ideas, the same words, the same sentence structure or at any rate, return to them again and again without any logical need."

The degree of perseverance of schizophrenic patients is similar to that of patients with known frontal pathology (Levin, 1984). Since Weinberger et al. (1986) reported a negative correlation between the percentage perseveration as measured by the Wisconsin Card Sorting Test, WCST, (Milner, 1963) and prefrontal blood flow, these associations have supported the hypothesis that schizophrenic patients have an impairment of the frontal or prefrontal cortex.

Because the clinical interpretation of test data can often point to multiple studies that converge on a set of frequent severe and selective deficits, patients with schizophrenia typically demonstrate abnormalities in attention, memory, and executive function that stand out against a background of diffuse impairment (Pantelis et al., 1996). However, some areas of function appear to be relatively more intact than others, i.e., some aspects of language (Gold et al., 1994; Saykin et al., 1991; Daniels et al., 1988; Barr et al., 1989; Frith, 1993) and some types of visual spatial processing (Kolb and Whishaw, 1983; Goldberg et al., 1990;

Goldberg et al., 1993a). These neuropsychological profiles implicate specific brain regions, i.e., frontal-medial dysfunction (Kolb and Whishaw, 1983; Taylor and Abrams, 1984). The finding that the aberration referred to functional body imageries would imply body image deficits that have some relation to dorsolateral deficits, and the fact that the anatomical, that is, visual and spatial, imageries remain intact is consistent with the previous finding that some types of visual spatial processing is intact in the neuropsychological profile of schizophrenics.

In Study 3, body image aberration was considered through an attempt to detect specific body image characteristics related to depression in schizophrenia by comparing the BIQ factor scores between depressive and non-depressive groups comprised by Zung's Self-rating Depression Scale (SDS) in normal and schizophrenic groups respectively. The results showed some body image factors related uniquely to depression in schizophrenia, which, again, referred to functional body images. The result of this part of the study might cast light on future prospects of the study of body image aberration using a device such as the BIQ because of its link with DSS which has become a target for treatment of schizophrenia, with the novel antipsychotic medications. The studies performed for this chapter all revealed that neuroleptics did not relate to body image aberration; however, novel antipsychotic agents were not discussed or studied. This would be relevant to the final question as to whether or not the body image aberration is remediable.

Study 4 and Study 5 are reports of subsidiary findings of our main studies using the BIQ, in which schizophrenic patients produced Rorschach responses implying or referring to "mass of flesh." Study 4 is composed of the initial observations. In Study 5, the Rorschach test was given to schizophrenic and non-schizophrenic subjects to determine whether schizophrenic patients more frequently produced the "mass of flesh" percept than the non-schizophrenic groups did. These findings suggest that there might be a fear of immobility in schizophrenia that is congruent with our main findings.

Conclusion

Schizophrenic body image aberration was considered in the current context. The schizophrenic body image aberration was unrelated to symptoms, insight, or conventional neuroleptic medication, but proved to be germane to schizophrenia. The schizophrenic body image aberration also proved to be limited to functional imagery while anatomical imageries remained intact.

Acknowledgments

We would like to express our appreciation to Dr. Chin-Piao Chien, professor emeritus of UCLA, and Dr. Shoji Shin'ichi and Dr. Susumu Oda, professors emeriti of Tsukuba University. We also thank Dr. Toshihiko Maeda of tne Institute of Statistical Mathematics for the statistical consultation.

Part of the text was re-edited from *Psychiatry and Clinical Neurosciences*, Vol. 56, pp9-15, "Body image, symptoms and insight in chronic schizophrenia" by Koide et al (2002), with permission from Blackwell Publishing, and from *Comprehensive Psychiatry,* Vol.43, pp474-477, "A mass of flesh: Schizophrenic Rorschach Percepts" by Koide R., et al (2002), with permission from Elsevier.

PART V. UPDATING SCHIZOPHRENIC BODY IMAGE DEVIATION: TOWARDS EARLY DETECTION OF SCHIZOPHRENIA IN ADOLESCENCE

In previous sections, we reported the schizophrenic body image as having a functional deviation and the body becoming perceived as an immovable mass. In this part, we attempted to apply the results of our findings to the diagnosis of schizophrenia in adolescence. In study 6, we show the results of the statistical analysis of the Body Image Questionnaire (BIQ) data obtained from male and female adolescent schizophrenia patients and age-matched controls, which were reported previously (Koide 1985, Baba and Koide 1989). In study 7, we report the cases of four adolescent who had seen Rorschach flesh masses (FMs) 1 to 8 years before the definite diagnosis of the disease was made. In this part, we attempt to apply the results of our findings for the diagnosis of schizophrenia in adolescents.

Study 6. BIQ Profiles in Adolescent Schizophrenia

Introduction

We re-analyzed the BIQ data obtained from adolescent schizophrenia patients and their age-matched controls between 1982 and 1989. The purpose of this study was to examine whether the body image deviation specific to schizophrenia obtained from the data analysis of chronic schizophrenic patients had also been observed in their youth.

Method

The schizophrenic group included 28 female schizophrenics aged 18 to 25, and the male schizophrenic group included 28 male schizophrenics aged 19 to 28. All of them had at least finished high school. Five females and 5 males had exhibited the first signs of schizophrenic symptoms within the previous five years. All of them were diagnosed with schizophrenia by two psychiatrists. The normal control group consisted of 30 female and 25 male college students aged 18 to 25. All of them were well-adapted to their school lives.

Results

Comparison between female groups

Statistically meaningful differences between female schizophrenic and female normal groups were found on 9 items. As shown in Table 15, female schizophrenics saw body images that were poorly proportioned, rough, unattractive, and having unusually short hair, indicating that they have an unattractive body image. Also, they reported images as being unable to move freely and having weak teeth, indicating negative images of body function. Also, it is noted that they saw images as becoming healthier, indicating strong hope that while their body (health) is now in bad condition, it will improve.

Table 15. Differences between means of female adolescent schizophrenic and normal groups

BIQ items	Group with higher mean
20. I am poorly proportioned.	S*
22. I seldom feel tired.®	S*
24. My body is rough.	S**
32. My body is unattractive.	S*
40. My hands are not unusually large.	N*
4I. I cannot move my body freely.	S**
46. My health is getting better. ®	N**
47. My teeth are weak.	S*
58. My hair is unusually short.	S*

* $p<0.05$, ** $p<0.01$, *** $p<0.001$

Comparison between male groups

As shown in Table 16, seven items statistically significantly differentiated male schizophrenic and control groups. Male schizophrenics saw body images as being tall, big, having good posture, and always appearing energetic. These results showed that young male schizophrenics saw more attractive body images compared to normal controls. However, they saw images of their body (health) as being becoming healthier, indicating a strong hope to overcome their bad body conditions, which were masked by extremely attractive images. They also saw body images as moving slowly (negative functional image).

Table 16. Differences between means of male adolescent schizophrenic and normal groups

BIQ items	Group with higher mean
08. I am short.	N**
09. I move slowly	S*
16. My body is small.	N*
33. My posture is good. ®	N*
40. My hands are not unusually large.	N*
46. My health is getting better. ®	N**

59. I always feel energetic.®	N**

* p<0.05, **p<0.01, ***p<0.001

Discussion and conclusion

The above results showed that, in adolescence, schizophrenics have a strong concern about the attractiveness of their bodies, which was not observed in chronic schizophrenia. This primary concern is reflected in their body images in two different ways in the different sexes. In women, it was reflected in seeing unattractive body images, while, in men, it was reflected in emphasizing their attractiveness. However, it is important that the body image of functionally declining and becoming immobilized is clearly observed in both sexes, although concern about the attractiveness of their body was prominent.

Study 7. Longitudinal Observation of Adolescent Cases Showing Rorschach Flesh Mass Responses

Introduction

We report four cases aged 19 to 23 years old that saw flesh mass responses and then developed obvious schizophrenic symptoms within 1 to 8 years. The purpose of this study is to confirm that observation of FMs can be one of the markers for a future diagnosis of schizophrenia.

Case Reports

Case E

Mr. E was a 19-year-old man when we administered the Rorschach test and found an MF. He was the oldest child of a garbage collector. He finished high school and got a job in a factory near his house. When he was 19, he suddenly withdrew from the workplace and stayed home all day. His supervisor took him to the hospital. E denied having hallucinations or delusions. He only complained of the severe noise in the factory. He explained to his doctor, "I just left my workplace to get away from the noise because it is so noisy, it makes me sick." He was suspected of schizophrenia. He was administered the Rorschach test and saw an FM. Atypical antipsychotic agent (olanzapine) was prescribed. After 6 months, he returned to the workplace. When he was 27 years old, he decided to live independently from his parents and moved to an apartment, but he soon complained that the neighbors were looking into his room. One day, he told his supervisor that he wanted to take leave to go to an exhibition of rifles that was being held the next day outside of town. His doctor persuaded him to take leave for a while to rest at home. After one year's leave, he returned to the factory, but he could no longer write simple documents properly nor discriminate items for picking packages in his workplace.

His FM response was to card I. "Two or three bats, clinging together."

Case F

Mr. F was a 23-year-old man when a Rorschach FM response was found. He was the oldest son of an executive officer of the government. He graduated from a university where he specialized in technology. After graduation at the age of 22, he was employed by a big company as an engineer. However, soon after employment, he began to take leave every two or three days complaining of a variety of physical symptoms, headache, backache, toothache, a ringing in his ears, stomachache, disturbance of his eyesight, fever, and so on. He visited many doctors, but no abnormality was found in the physical examinations. He went the office but did not work, complaining of one physical condition after another. One year later, when he was 23, he complained of being woken up every day by nightmares in which he was being pursued by somebody. His supervisor noticed that he did not go out for lunch. He explained to the supervisor, "The bad dreams are frightening, but they are just dreams." He also said "I cannot eat out because it is my custom since childhood to eat only foods my family has cooked for me." He was taken to a psychiatrist, but the doctor did not recognize hallucination or delusion. He suspected schizophrenia, and prescribed atypical antipsychotics (risperidone). A Rorschach FM response was observed at the first visit to the psychiatric clinic. After 2 years' leave, he returned to the office. His supervisor noticed that he could then eat in restaurants, but no longer perform the job of an engineer.

His FM response was to card III. "Birds and animals are clinging together to a tree, as if they make a small mass."

Case G

Mr. G was 23-year-old man, when a Rorschach FM response was observed. He was the first son of the owner of a small shop. He graduated from university specializing in technology and was employed by a company as an engineer at the age of 22. He was highly evaluated after employment by the other staff members, but when he was 23, he suddenly traveled 1000 km from his working place. He said that his family was in danger. He thought that somebody was talking ill of him on the internet, so could not leave his computer and watched it all day. He was brought to the hospital by his parents and was admitted. He was suspected of schizophrenia and medicated with olanzapine. Soon after admission, positive psychotic symptoms disappeared, and the Rorschach test was administered. He returned to the office after one year's leave, but his superior complained that he did not work as well as before. He forgot directions from his supervisor, worked slowly, lost documents, and often left the workplace to wander around the company.

His FM response was to card X. "Dancing. ([Examiner] Can you identify what is dancing?) It is not clear, however, I guess something like human beings, or dwarfs. These red parts are heads, here. No arms. No legs."

Case H

Miss H was a 22-year-old woman when she observed a Rorschach FM. She was the third child of the family of a businessman. She graduated from college, specializing in technology.

Four months after employment, she complained that she felt as if she was being pressed by people around her, left the office, visited a doctor who administered the Rorschach test. She returned to work after one year's leave, but she complained that other staff members talked ill of her and left the office again. She said, "I feel like that people around me say that married women are different from those who are not married."

Her FM response was to card IV. "Some strange animals without legs or arms fixed together."

Discussion and Conclusion

These four cases were administered the Rorschach test when the first sign of schizophrenia was shown, and the diagnoses of schizophrenia were made later. Three of them were medicated with atypical antipsychotics. The first psychotic experiences of cases E and F were modified and sophisticated: denying hallucination and complaining of mere noise in the factory in the case of E, and the delusion of being poisoned by food was transformed into a desire to eat his childhood foods and a feeling of persecution was recognized as it happened in the dream in the case of F. In Cases G and H, the psychotic experience occurred once and soon disappeared, but recurred again. In all four cases, a FM was observed in the phase before the diagnoses were definitely made.

Conclusion

Onset of schizophrenia in adolescence is quite common. However, it often takes years of observation to make a definite diagnosis. In some cases, psychotic symptoms such as hallucinations and delusions are covered by sophisticated talk or behavior or modified by physical complaints, which make accurate diagnosis quite difficult. In most cases, physicians may suspect schizophrenia, but they need to observe the progress of the disease to make the diagnosis of schizophrenia.

In previous parts of this chapter, we discussed the body image deviation characteristic of schizophrenia as a deviant functional or immovable body image, which is detected in chronic schizophrenia. In this part, we considered whether this characteristic is also observed in schizophrenia in adolescence. As shown above, body image deviation in body function was also observed in young schizophrenics.

In the BIQ, the functional items differentiated schizophrenic and control groups at a statistically significant level. Also, schizophrenic groups of both sexes were shown to be hopeful about their body ("My health is getting better"), reflecting their bad physical condition. Although it is commonly thought that physical attractiveness is the first concern of the young, deviant images of body function are obviously observed in adolescent schizophrenia, although they are masked by primary concern about their attractiveness.

We showed cases in which we could observe the progress of schizophrenia for 1 to 8 years after FM responses were found, when schizophrenia was suspected, but not obviously diagnosed, by a psychiatrist. Although these responses were found to be characteristic not only of chronic but also of acute schizophrenia in previous sections, observation of these four cases show the effectiveness of these responses in the diagnosis of schizophrenia prior to the clear onset of the disease when psychotic symptoms are manifested.

The facts reported here suggest the possibility that we can use the body image deviation reported in this chapter as one of the markers to detect schizophrenia in its early phase in adolescence.

Appendix

Appendix 1. Manual for Scoring the Body Image Questionnaire

Appendix 1-1. Overview of the Questionnaire and the Scoring System

Reverse items The BIQ is composed of 59 items, including 28 reverse questions. Reverse items are Nos. 2, 4, 7, 12, 13, 14, 15, 22, 26, 27, 28, 30, 31, 33, 35, 36, 37, 38, 42, 43, 44, 46, 48, 50, 52, 55, 57 and 59.

Scoring system In *Regular items*, answers are scored as 7 when one "strongly agrees" with the statements, and scored as 1 when one "strongly disagrees" to the statements. In the *Reverse items*, answers are scored as 1 when one "strongly agrees" with the statements, and scored as 7 when one "strongly disagrees" with the statements. Answers as "neither agree nor disagree" are scored as 4.

BIQ component BIQ has three Components, Anatomical, Functional and Psychological. *Anatomical items* are Nos. 4, 8, 15, 16, 18, 20, 24, 28, 36, 40, 44, 48, 52, 54, 55, 56, 57 and 58. (See Apendix 1-3.) *Functional items* are: Nos. 1, 2, 3, 5, 9, 13, 17, 21, 25, 33, 37, 38, 41, 42, 47 and 53. (See Appendix 1-4.) *Psychological items* are Nos. 6, 7, 10, 11, 12, 14, 19, 22, 23, 26, 27, 29, 30, 31, 32, 34, 35, 39, 43, 45, 46, 49, 50, 51 and 59. (See Appendix 1-5.)

Appendix 1-2. Body Image Questionnaire (BIQ)

	Strongly disagree	Moderately disagree	Slightly agree	Neither agree nor disagree	Slightly agree	Moderately agree	Strongly agree
01. My body is weak.							
02. My eyesight is good. ®							
03. I often get sick.							
04. My complexion is pale. ®							
05. My body is limber.							

	Strongly disagree						
06. My body is underdeveloped.							
07. My body is clean.®							

Appendix 1-2. (Continued)

08. I am short.							
09. I move slowly							
10. My body is defective.							
11. My body feels cold.							
12. My body is beautiful.®							
13. I am good at athletics.®							
14. I am becoming stronger. ®							
15. My body is skinny. ®							
16. My body is small.							
17. I often lose my balance.							
18. I have small eyes.							
19. I am often injured.							
20. I am poorly proportioned.							
21. I walk slowly.							
22. I seldom feel tired.®							
23. My mood is numb.							
24. My body is rough.							
25. I am clumsy with my hands.							
26. I seldom catch a cold.®							
27. I am satisfied with my body. ®							
28. I am thin.®							
29. My voice is feeble.							
30. My skin is not easily poisoned. ®							
31. I am always cheerful. ®							
32. My body is unattractive.							
33. My posture is good. ®							
34. I always feel sick.							
35. I am not allergic to many things. ®							
36. My skin is smooth.®							
37. I can work well in dark rooms. ®							
38. My stomach is not unusually strong. ®							
39. My body is susceptible to infection.							
40. My hands are not unusually large.							
4I. I cannot move my body freely.							
42. My heart is strong. ®							
43. I don’t mind being touched by others. ®							
44. My body is not meager.®							
45. I seldom get excited.							

46. My health is getting better. ®							
47. My teeth are weak.							
48. My body is symmetrical.®							
49. I am seldom tense.							
50. I am not prone to bump into others. ®							

Appendix 1-2. (Continued)

51. My body is not consistent with my sex.							
52. My body is rectangular. ®							
53. My bowels are unusually strong.							
54. My legs are unusually short.							
55. My arms are unusually long. ®							
56. My neck is unusually long.							
57. My head is large. ®							
58. My hair is unusually short.							
59. I always feel energetic.®							

®=reverse item.

Appendix 1-3. BIQ-Anatomical items

04. My complexion is pale. ®
08. I am short.
15. My body is skinny. ®
16. My body is small.
18. I have small eyes.
20. I am poorly proportioned.
24. My body is rough.
28. I am thin. ®
36. My skin is smooth. ®
40. My hands are not unusually large.
44. My body is not meager. ®.
48. My body is symmetrical. ®.
52. My body is rectangular. ®
54. My legs are unusually short.
55. My arms are unusually long. ®
56. My neck is unusually long.
57. My head is large. ®
58. My hair is unusually short.

®=reverse item.

Appendix 1-4. BIQ-Functional items

01. My body is weak.
02. My eyesight is good. ®

03. I often get sick.
05. My body is limber.
09. I move slowly
13. I am good at athletics.®
17. I often lose my balance.
21. I walk slowly.

Appendix 1-4. (Continued)

25. I am clumsy with my hands.
33. My posture is good. ®
37. I can work well in dark rooms. ®
38. My stomach is not unusually strong. ®
41. I cannot move my body freely.
42. My heart is strong. ®
47. My teeth are weak.
53. My bowels are unusually strong.

®=reverse item.

Appendix 1-5. BIQ Psychological items

06. My body is underdeveloped.
07. My body is clean. ®
10. My body is defective.
11. My body feels cold.
12. My body is beautiful. ®
14. I am becoming stronger. ®
19. I am often injured.
22. I seldom feel tired. ®
23. My mood is numb.
26. I seldom catch a cold. ®
27. I am satisfied with my body. ®
29. My voice is feeble.
30. My skin is not easily poisoned. ®
31. I am always cheerful. ®
32. My body is unattractive.
34. I always feel sick.
35. I am not allergic to many things. ®
39. My body is susceptible to infection.
43. I don't mind being touched by others. ®
45. I seldom get excited.
46. My health is getting better. ®
49. I am seldom tense.
50. I am not prone to bump into others. ®
51. My body is not consistent with my sex.

59. I always feel energetic.®

Appendix 2. Inclusion and exclusion criteria for perception of flesh masses

Inclusion
1. Explicit verbalization of a mass of flesh or muscles.
2. The remains of a mass of flesh.
3. Diminution of head, arm or leg.
4. Elongation of neck, arm or leg.
5. Plants or vehicles described as "without arms or legs.[1]"
6. A creature with the shape of a mass[2].
7. A single organ vaguely detected with no further explanation.
8. "Being cut and opened," "being folded," "being unfolded," or "being stuck together".
Exclusion
1. Underdeveloped animals or human beings, or animals that have intrinsically short arms or legs, without further explanation concerning diminution of arms or legs.
2. Omission of legs in the response to Card VII.

Note: 1. Examples are: "A tropical flower. I cannot find its arms or legs." "An airplane. It doesn't have any arms or legs." 2. Example is: "A prawn. It is in this globular shape, with his back hunching up in this way."

References

Amador, X. F., Flaum, M,, Andreasen, N.C., Strauss, D. H., Yale, S. A., Clark, S. C. and Gorman, J. M. (1994). Awareness of illness in schizophrenia and schizoaffective and Mood disorders. *Archives of General Psychiatry, 51*, 826-836.

Amador, X. F., Strauss, D.H., Yale, S.A., and Gorman JM. (1991). Awareness of illness in schizophrenia. *Schizophrenia Bulletin, 17*,113-132.

American Psychiatric Association. (1980). *Diagnostic and statistical manual of mental disorders (3rd edition)*. Washington, DC: American Psychiatric Association.

American Psychiatric Association. (1987). *Diagnostic and statistical manual of mental disorders (3rd edition revised)*. Washington, DC: American Psychiatric Association.

American Psychiatric Association. (1994). *Diagnostic and statistical manual of mental disorders (4th edition)*. Washington, DC: American Psychiatric Association.

Andreasen, N. C. (1981). *Scale for the assessment of negative symptoms*. Iowa City, IA: The University of Iowa Press.

Andreasen, N. C. (1983). *Scale for the assessment of positive symptoms*. Iowa City, IA: The University of Iowa Press.

Andreasen, N. C., Arndt, S., Alliger, R., Miller, D., and Flaum, M. (1995). Symptoms of schizophrenia: methods, meanings, and mechanisms. *Archives of General Psychiatry, 52*, 341-351.

Andreasen, N, and Bardach, J. (1977). Dysmorphophobia:Symptom or disease? *American Journal of Psychiatry, 134*, 673-676.

Angyal, A. (1936). Experiences of body self in schizophrenia. *Archives of Neurology and Psychiatry, 35*, 1629-1634.

Apter, J.T. (1981). The "silent" acute abdomen in schizophrenia. *Journal of the Medical Society of New Jersey, 78*, 679-680.

Arieti, S. (1945). Primitive habits and perceptual alterations in the terminal stage of schizophrenia. *Archives of Neurology and Psychiatry, 53*, 378-384.

Baba, K., Koide, R. (1989). Body image deviation in male schizophrenia. Annuals of Liberal Arts, University of Gunnma, 39, 291-300. (In Japanese.)

Barr, W. B., Bilder, R. M., Goldberg, E. H., Caplan, E., and Mukherjee, S. (1989). The neuropsychology of schizophrenic speech. *Journal of Communication Disorders, 22*, 327-349.

Berman, A. L. (1972). Videotape self-confrontation of schizophrenic ego and thought processes. *Journal of Consulting and Clinical Psychology, 39,* 78-85.

Bickerstaff, L. K., Harris, S. C, Leggett R S, and Cheah K. C. (1988). Pain insensitivity in schizophrenic patients: A surgical dilemma. *Archives of Surgery, 123*, 49-50.

Bilder, R. M., and Goldberg, R. E. (1987) Motor perseverations in schizoiphrenia. *Archives of Clinical Neuropsychology, 2*, 195-214.

Birtchnell, S. A. (1988). Dysmorphophobia - a centenary discussion. *British Journal of Psychiatry, 153 (suppl 2)*, 41-43.

Blackmore, S. (1986). Out-of-body experiences in schizophrenia. A questionnaire survey. *Journal of Nervous and Mental Disease, 174*, 615-619.

Bleuler, E. (1911) *Dementia Praecox, or the Group of Schizophrenias*. Translated by J Zinkin. New York: International Universities Press (1950).

Braff, D. L., Heaton, R., Kuck, J., Cullum, M., Moranville, J., Grant, I., and Zisook, S. (1991). The generalized pattern of neuropsychological deficits in outpatients with chronic schizophrenia with heterogeneous Wisconsin Card Sorting Test results. *Archives of General Psychiatry, 158*, 340-345.

Brebion, G., Smith, M. J., Amador, X., Malaspina, D., and Gorman, J.M. (1997). Clinical correlates of memory in schizophrenia: differential links between depression, positive and negative symptoms, and two types of memory impairment. *American Journal of Psychiatry, 154*, 1538-1543.

Bryson, G., Bell, M., Lysaker, P. (1997). Affect recognition in schizophrenia: A function of global impairment or a specific cognitive deficit. *Psychiatry Research, 71*, 105-113.

Buchanan, R. W., Strauss, M. E., Breier, A., Kirkpatrick, B., and Carpenter, W.T. (1997). Attentional impairements in deficit and nondeficit forms of schizophrenia. *American Journal of Psychiatry, 154*, 363-370.

Burgess, J. W. (1991). Relationship of depression and cognitive impairment to self-injury in borderline personality disorder, major depression, and schizophrenia. *Psychiatry Research, 38*, 77-87.

Bychowsky, G. (1943). Disorders of the body image in the clinical picture of psychoses. *Journal of Nerveous and Mental Disease, 97*, 310-334.

Caldwell, C. B., and Gottesman, I.I. (1990). Schizophrenics kill themselves too: a review of risk factors for suicide. *Schizophrenia Bulletin, 16*, 571-589.

Cancro, R. (1971). Sophistication of body concept in process-reactive schizophrenia. *Perceptual and Motor Skills, 32*, 567-570.

Cassens, G., Inglis, A. K., Appelbaum, P. S., and Gutheil, T. G. (1990). Neuroleptics: Effects on neuropsychological function in chronic schizophrenic patients. *Schizophrenia Bulletin, 16*, 477-499.

Censits, D. M., Ragland, J. D., Gur, R. C., and Gur, R. E. (1997). Neuropsychological evidence supporting a neurodevelopmental model of schizophrenia: A longitudinal study. *Schizophrenia Research, 24*, 289-298.

Chapman, L. J., Chapman, J.P., and Raulin, M. L. (1976). Scales for physical and social anhedonia. *Journal of Abnormal Psychology, 85*, 374-382.

Chapman, L. J., Chapman, J. P., and Raulin, M. L. (1978). Body-image aberration in schizophrenia. *Journal of Abnormal Psychology, 87*, 399-407.

Cleveland, S. E. (1960a). Body image changes associated with personality reorganization. *Journal of Consulting Psychology, 24*, 256-261.

Cleveland, S. E. (1960b). Judgements of body size in a schizophrenic and a control group. *Psychological Reports, 7*, 304.

Cleveland, S. E., Fisher, S., Reitman, E. E., and Rothaus, P. (1962). Perception of body size in schizophrenia. *Archives of General Psychiatry, 7*, 277-285.

Cohen, L. J., Test, M. A. and Brocon, R. L. (1990). Suicide and schizophrenia: data from a prospective community treatment study. *American Journal of Psychiatry, 147*, 602-607. Correction, 147, 1110.

Coleman, M. J., Carpenter, J. T., Waterneaux, C., Levy, D. L., Shenton, M. E., Perry, J., Medoff, D., Wong, H., Manoach, D., Meyer, P., O'Brien, C., Valentino, C., Robinson, D., Smith, M., Makowski, D. and Holzman, P. S. (1993) The Thought Disorder Index: A reliability study. *Psychological Assessment, 5*, 336-342.

Coleman, M. J., Levy, D. L., Lenzenweger, M. F. and Holzman, P. S. (1996) Thought disorder, perceptual aberrations, and schizotypy. *Journal of Abnormal Psychology, 105*, 469-473.

Connolly, F. and Gipson, M. (1978). Dysmorphophobia. A long term study. *British Journal of Psychiatry, 132*, 458-470.

Coons, P. M., Ascher-Svanum, H, and Bellis, K. (1986). Self-amputation of the female breast. *Psychosomatics, 27*, 667-668.

Cornblatt, B. A., Lenzenweger, M. F., Dworkin, R. H. and Erlenmeyer-Kimling, L. (1985). Positive and negative schizophrenic symptoms, attention, and information processing. *Schizophrenia Bulletin, 11*, 397-408.

Crider, A. (1997). Perseverations in schiziophrenia. *Schizophrenia Bulletin, 23*, 63-74.

Crow, T. J. and Johnstone, E. C. (1980). Dementia praecox and schizophrenia: was Bleuler wrong? *Journal of the Royal College of Physicians, 14*, 238-240.

Crow, T. J. and Stevens, M. (1978). Age disorientation in chronic schizophrenia: the nature of the cognitive deficit. *British Journal of Psychiatry, 133*, 137-142.

Cuesta, M. J. and Peralta, V. (1994). Lack of insight in schizophrenia. *Schizophrenia Bulletin, 20*, 359-366.

Cuesta, M. S., Peralta, V., Caro, F, and de Leon, J. (1995). Schizophrenia syndrome and Wisconsin Card Sorting Test dimensions. *Psychiatry Research, 58*, 45-51.

Daniels, E. K., Shenton, M. E., Holzman, P. S., Benowitz, L. I., Coleman, M. ,Levin, S. and Levine, D. (1988). Patterns of thought disorder associated with right cortical damage, schizophrenia, and mania. *American Journal of Psychiatry, 145*, 944-949.

Darby, J. A. (1968). Pychotheraputic treatment of schizophrenia: Theory and case study. *Psychotherapy: Theory, Research, and Practice, 5*, 234-239.

David, S. A. (1990). Insight and psychosis. *British Journal of Psychiatry, 156*, 798-808.

Delaplaine, R., Ifabumuyi, O. I., Merskey, H. and Zarfas, J. (1978). Significance of pain in psychiatirc hospital patients. *Pain, 4*, 361-366.

deLeon, J., Bott, A. and Simpson, G. H. (1989). Dysmorphophobia: body dysmorphic disorder or delusional disorder, somatic type? *Comprehensive Psychiatry, 30*, 457-472.

Des Lauriers, A. M. (1962). *The experience of reality in childhood schizophrenia.* New York: International Universities Press.

Dillon, D. J. (1962) Measurement of perceived body size. *Perceptual and Motor Skills,14*, 191-196.

Dingman, C. W. and McGlashan, T. H. (1986). Discriminating characteristics of suicides: Chestnut Lodge follow-up sample including patients with affective disorder, schizophrenia and schizoaffective disorder. *Acta Psychiatrica Scandinavica, 74*, 91-97.

Dingman, C. W. and McGlaschan, T. H. (1988). Characteristics of patients with serious suicidal inpatients who ultimately commit suicide. *Hospital and Community Psychiatry, 39*, 295-299.

Di-Nuovo, S., Laicardi, C. and Tobino, C. (1988). Rorschach indices for discriminating between two schizophrenic syndromes. *Perceptual and Motor Skills, 67*, 399-406.

Drake, R. E. and Cotton, P. G. (1986). Depression, hopelessness and suicide in chronic schizophrenia. *British Journal of Psychiatry, 148*, 554-559.

Dworkin, R. H. (1994). Pain insensitivity in schizophrenia: A neglected phenomenon and some implications. *Schizophrenia Bulletin, 20*, 235-248.

Dworkin, R. H. and Caligor, E. (1988). Psychiatric diagnosis and chronic pain: DSM III-R and beyond. *Journal of Pain and Symptom Management, 3*, 87-98.

Edgerton, M., Jacobsen, W. and Meyer, E. (1960) Surgical/ psychiatric study of patients seeking plastic (cosmetic) surgery: 98 consecutive patients with minimal deformity. *British Journal of Plastic Surgery, 13*, 136-145.

Exner, E. J. Jr. (1974). *The Rorschach: A Comprehensive System: Vol.1*. Basic Foundations. New York: Wiley.

Exner, E. J. Jr. (1978). *The Rorschach: A Comprehensive System: Vol.2*. Current Research and Advanced Interpretation. New York: Wiley.

Exner, E. J. Jr. (1986a). *The Rorschach: A Comprehensive System: Vol.1*. Basic Foundations. 2nd ed. New York: Wiley.

Exner, E. J. Jr. (1986b). Some Rorschach data comparing schizophrenics with borderline and schizotypal personality disorders. *Journal of Personality Assessment, 50*, 455-471.

Exner, E. J. Jr. (1991). *The Rorschach: A Comprehensive System: Vol.2*. Current Research and Advanced Interpretation. 2nd ed. New York: Wiley.

Exner EJ Jr. (1993). *The Rorschach: A Comprehensive System: Vol.1*. Basic Foundations (3rd edition). New York: Wiley.

Federn P. (1952). *Ego Psychology and the psychosis*. New York: Basic Books.

Feldman MD. 1988 The challenge of self-mutilation: a review. *Comprehensive Psychiatry, 29*, 252-269.

Ferenczi, S. (1926). The problem of acceptance of unpleasant ideas: Advances in knowledge of the sense of reality. *International Journal of Psychoanalysis, 7*, 312-323.

Fishbain, D. A. (1982) Pain insensitivity in psychosis. *Annals of Emergency Medicine, 11*, 630-632.

Fisher, S. (1963). A further appraisal of the body boundary concept. *Journal of Consulting Psychology, 27*, 62-74.

Fisher, S. (1964). Body image and psychopathology. *Archives of General Psychiatry, 10*, 519-529.

Fisher, S. (1966). Body image in neurotic and schizophrenic patients. *Archives of General Psychiatry, 15*, 90-101.

Fisher, S. and Cleveland, S. E. (1958). *Body image and personality*. Princeton, NJ; Van Nostrand.

Fisher, S. and Cleveland S. E. (1968). *Body image and personality 2nd edition)*. New York: Dover Publications.

Fisher, S. and Renik, O.D. (1966). Induction of body image boundary changes. *Journal of Projective Techniques and Personality Assessment, 30*, 429-434.

Fisher, S. and Seidner, R. (1963). Body experiences of schizophrenic, neurotic and normal women. *Journal of Nervous and Mental Disease, 137*, 252-257.

Fottrell, E. (1980). A study of violent behaviour among patients in psychiatric hospitals. *British Journal of Psychiatry, 136*, 216-221.

Freeman, T., Cameron, J. L. and McGhie, A. (1958). *Chronic Schizophrenia*. New York: International Universities Press.

Freeman, T. and Gathercole, L. E. (1966). Perseveration in chronic schizophrenia and organic dementia. *British Journal of Psychiatry, 112*, 27-32.

Freud, S. (1962). *The ego and the id*. New York: Norton.

Frith, C. (1993). *The Cognitive Neuropsychology of Schizophrenia*. Erlbaum, Hove.

Galdi, J. (1983). The causality of depression in schizophrenia. *British Journal of Psychiatry, 142*, 621-624.

George, L. and Neufeld, R. W. (1985). Cognition and symptomatology in schizophrenia. *Schizophrenia Bulletin, 11*, 264-285.

Gerstmann, J. (1942). Problem of imperception of disease and of impaired body territories with organic lesions. Relation to body schema and its disorders. *Archives of Neurology and Psychiatry, 48*, 890-913.

Gold, J. M., Hermann, B.P., Wyler, A., Randolph, C., Goldberg, T.E. and Weinberger, D. R. (1994). Schizophrenia and temporal lobe epilepsy: a neuropsychological study. *Archives of General Psychiatry, 51*, 265-272.

Goldberg, D. P. (1972). *The detection of psychiatric illness by questionnaire*. Maudsley Monograph 21. London: Oxford University Press.

Goldberg, D. and Williams, P. (1988). *A user's guide to the General Health Questionnaire*. Windsor, Berkshire: Neer-Nelson.

Goldberg, T. E., Gold, J. M., Greenberg, R., Griffin, S., Schulz, S. C., Picker, D., Kleinman, J. E., and Weinberger, D. R. (1993a). Contrasts between patients with affective disorder and patients with schizophrenia on a neuropsychological screening test battery. *American Journal of Psychiatry, 150*, 1355-1362.

Goldberg, T. E., Greenberg, R. and Griffin, S. (1993b). The impact of clozapine on cognition and psychiatric symptoms in patients with schizophrenia. *British Journal of Psychiatry, 162*, 43-48.

Goldberg, T.E., Ragland, D.R., Gold, J., Bigelow, L.B., Torrey, E.F. and Weinberger, D. R. (1990). Neuropsychological assessment of monozygotic twins discordant for schizophrenia. *Archives of General Psychiatry 47*, 1066-1072.

Goldstein, G. (1978). Cognitive and perceptual differences between schizophrenics and organics. *Schizophrenia Bulletin, 4*, 160-185.

Goodenough, F. L. (1928). Studies in the psychology of children's drawings. *Psychological Bulletin, 25*, 272-279.

Green, M. F. (1996). What are the functional consequences of neurocognitive deficit in schizophrenia? *American Journal of Psychiatry, 153*, 321-330.

Green, M. F., Marshall, B. D., Wirshing, W. C., Ames, D., Marder, S. R., McGurk, S., Kern, R. S. and Mintz, J. (1997). Does risperidone improve verbal working mempry in treatment–resistant schizophrenia? *American Journal of Psychiatry, 154*, 799-804.

Green, M. F. and Nuechterlein, K. H. (1999). Should schizophrenia be treated as a neurocognitive disorder? *Schizophrenia Bulletin, 25*, 309-318.

Green, M. F., Nuechterlein, K. H. and Geier, D.J. (1992). Sustained and selective attention in schizophrenia. *Progress in Experimental Personaity and Psychopathology Research, 15*, 290-313.

Green, M. F. and Walker, E. (1985). Neuropsychological performance and positive and negative symptoms in schizophrenia. *Journal of Abnormal Psychology, 94*, 460-469.

Guieu, R., Samuelian, J. C. and Coulouvrat, H. (1994). Objective evaluation of pain perception in patients with schizophrenia. *British Journal of Psychiatry, 164*, 253-255.

Hagger, C., Buckley, P., Kenny, J. T., Friedman, L., Ubogy, D. and Meltzer, H. Y. (1993). Improvement in cognitive functions and psychiatric symptoms in treatment –refractory schizopherenic patients receiving clozapine. *Bioliogical Psychiatry, 34*, 702-712.

Harding, C. M., Zubin, J. and Strauss, S. (1992). Chronicity in schizophrenia. *British Journal of Psychiatry, 161 (Suppl 18)*, 27-37.

Hay, G. (1970). Dysmorphophobia. *British Journal of Psychiatry, 116*, 399-406.

Hay, G. (1973). Changes in psychometric test results following cosmetic nasal operations. *British Journal of Psychiatry, 122*, 89-90.

Hay, G. (1983). Paranoia and dysmorphophobia. *British Journal of Psychiatry, 142*, 309-310.

Head, H. (1911). Sensory disturbunce from cerebral lesions. *Brain, 34*, 187-189.

Head, H. (1926). *Aphasia and Kindred Disorders of Speech*. London: Cambridge University Press.

Heaton, R. K., Baade, L. E. and Johnson, K. L. (1978). Neuropsychological test results associated with psychiatric disorders in adults. *Psychological Bulletin, 85*,141-162.

Hill, G. and Silver, G. (1950). Psychodynamics and esthetic motivations for plastic surgery. *Psychosomatic Medicine, 12*, 345-355.

Hilsenroth, M. J., Fowler, J. C. and Padawer, J. R. (1998). The Rorschach Schizophrenia Index (SCZI): an examination of reliability, validity, and diagnostic efficacy. *Journal of Personality Assessment, 70*, 514-534.

Himelhoch, S., Taylor, S. F., Goldman, R. S. and Tandon, R. (1996). Frontal lobes, antipsychotic medication, and schizophrenic symptoms. *Biological Psychiatry, 39*, 227-229.

Hirsch, S. R. (1982). Depression "revealed" in schizophrenia. *British Journal of Psychiatry, 140*, 421-424.

Hollander, E., Cohen, L. T. and Simeon, D. (1993). Body dysmorphic disorder. *Psychiatric Annals, 23*, 359-364.

Holt, R. (1977). A method for assessing primary process manifestations and their controls in Rorschach responses. In M. Rickers-Ovsiankina (Eds), *Rorschach Psychology (2nd edition, pp375-420)*. Huntington, NY: Krieger.

Holtzman, W. H., Gorham, D. R. and Moran, L. J. (1964). A factor-analytic study of schizophrenic thought processes. *Journal of Abnormal and Social Psychology, 69*, 355-364.

Holtzman, W. H., Thorpe, J. S., Swartz, J. D. and Herron, E.W. (1961*). Inkblot perception and personality: Holtzman inkblot technique*. Austin: University of Texas Press.

Hu, W. H., Sun, C. M., Lee, C. T., Peng, S. L., Lin, S. K. and Shen, W. W. (1991). A clinical study of schizophrenic suicides: 42 cases in Taiwan. *Schizophrenia Research, 5,* 43-50.

Huber, G. (1957). Die coenaesthetische Schizophrenie. *Fortschritte der Neurologie und Psychiatrie, 25*, 491-520.

Huber, G. (1971). Die coenaesthetische Schizophrenie als Praegnanztyp schizophrener Erkrankungen. *Acta Psychiatrica Scandinavica, 47*, 349-362.

Humphreys, M. S., Johnstone, E. C., MacMillan, J. F. and Taylor, P. J. (1992). Dangerous behaviour preceding first admission s for schizophrenia. *British Journal of Psychiatry, 161*, 501-505.

Jacobsen, W., Edgerton, M., Meyer, E., Canter, A. and Slaughter, R. (1960). Psychiatric evaluation of male patients seeking cosmetic surgery. *Plastic and Reconstructive Surgery, 16*, 356-372.

Jasker, R. O. and Reed, M. R. (1963). Assessment of body image organization of hospitalizd and non-hopspitalized subjects. *Journal of Projective Techniques, 27*, 185-190.

Jeste, D. V., Lohr, J. B., Eastman, J. H., Rockwell, E. and Caligiuri, M. P. (1998). Adverse neurobiological effects of long term use of neuroleptics: Human and animal studies. *Journal of Psychiatric Research, 32*, 201-214.

Johnston, M, and Holzman, P. (1979). *Assessing Schizophrenic Thinking*. San Francisco: Jossey-Bass.

Johnstone, E. C., Crow, T. J., Frith, C. D., Husband, J. and kreel, L. (1976). Cerebral ventricular size and cognitive impairment in chronic schizophrenia. *Lancet II,* 924-926.

Katz, E., Kluger, Y., Rabinovici, R., Stein, D. and Gimmon, Z. (1990). Acute surgical abdominal disease in chronic svhizohrenic patients: A unique clinical problem. *Israel Journal of Medical Sciences, 26*, 275-277.

Kay, S. R., Fiszbein, A. and Opler, L.A. (1987). The positive and negative syndrome scale (PANSS) for schizophrenia. *Schizophrenia Bulletin, 13*, 261-276.

Keefe, R. S. E., Silva, S. G., Perkins, D. O. and Lieberman, J. A. (1999). The effects of atypical antipsychotic drugs on neurocognitive impairmaent in schizophrenia: A review and meta-analysis. *Schizophrenia Bulletin, 25*, 201-222.

Kennedy, B. L. and Feldmann, T. B. (1994). Self-inflicted eye injuries: case presentation s and a literature review. *Hospital Community Psychiatry, 45*, 470-474.

Kern, R. S., Green, M. F., Marshall, B. D., Wirshing, W. C., McGurk, S. R., Marder, S. R. and Mintz, J. (1999). Risperidone vs haloperidol on secondary memory: Can newer antipsychotic medications aid learning? *Schizophrenia Bulletin, 25*, 223-233.

Knights, A. and Hirsch, S. R. (1981). “Revealed” depression and drug treatment for schizophrenia. *Archives of General Psychiatry, 38*, 806-811.

Koide, R. (1985). Body image differences between schizophrenic and normal female adults. International *Review of Applied Psychology, 34*, 335-347.

Kokonis, N. D. (1972). Body image disturbance in schizophrenia. A study of arms and feet. *Journal of Personality Assessment, 36*, 573-575.

Kolb, B. and Whishaw, .IQ. (1983). Performance of schizophrenic patients on tests sensitive to left or right frontal temporal, and parietal function in neurologic patients. *Journal of Nervous and Mental Disease, 171*, 435-443.

Kraepelin, E. (1919). *Dementia Praecox and Paraphrenia*. Edinburgh, Scotland: E. and S. Livingstone.

Kuechenhoff, J. (1984).Dysmorphophobie. *Nervenarzt, 55*, 122-126.

Kwawer, J. (1980). Primitive interpersonal modes, borderline phenomena and Rorschach content. In J. Kwawer, H. Lerner, P. Lerner and A. Sugarman (Eds). *Borderline Phenomena and Rorschach Test* (pp. 257-274). New York: International University Press.

Lautenbacher, S. and Krieg, J. C. (1994). Pain perception in psychiatric disorders: a review of the literature. *Journal of Psychiatry Research, 28*, 109-122.

Leventhal, D. B., Schuck, J. R., Clemons, J. T. and Cox, M. (1982). Proprioception in schizophrenia. *Journal of Nervous and Mental Disease, 170*, 21-26.

Levin, S. (1984). Frontal lobe dysfunction in schizophrenia II. Impairments of psychological and brain functions. *Journal of Psychiatric Research, 18*, 27-55.

Liddle, P. F. and Morris, D.L. (1991). Schizophrenic syndromes and frontal lobe performance. *British Journal of Psychiatry, 158*, 340-345.

Linn, L. and Goldman, I. (1949). Psyciatric observations concerning rhinoplasty. *Psychosomatic Medicine, 11*, 307-309.

Lukianowicz, N. (1967). Body image disturbances in psychiatric disorders. *British Journal of Psychiatry, 113*, 31-47.

Lysaker, P. and Bell, M. (1994). Insight and cognitive impairment in schizophrenia: Performance on repeated administrations of the Wisconsin Card Sorting Test. *Journal of Nervous and Mental Disease, 182*, 656-660.

Machover, K. (1949). *Personality projection in the drawing of the human figure. Springfield, III.*: Chales C Thomas.

Malec, J. (1978). Neuropsychological assessment of schizophrenia versus brain damage: a review. *Journal of Nervous and Mental Disease, 166*, 507-516.

Manschreck, T. C., Maher, B. A., Hoover, T. M. and Ames D. (1985). Repetition in schizophrenic speech. *Language and Speech, 28*, 327-349.

Marchand, W. E. (1959). Practice of surgery in a neuropsychiatric hospital. *Archives of General Psychiatry, 1*, 123-131.

Martin, R. L., Cloninger, C. R. and Guze, S. B. (1985). Frequency and differetial diagnosis of depressive syndromes in schizophrenia. *Journal of Clinical Psychiatry, 46*, 9-13.

Martin, T. and Gattaz, W. F. (1991). Psychiatric aspects of male genital self-mutilation. *Psychopathology, 24*, 170-178.

Mason, B., Cohen, J. and Exner, J. E. Jr. (1985). Schizophrenic, depressive, and nonpatient personality organizations described by Rorschach factor structures. *Journal of Personality Assessment, 49*, 295-305.

Mayer-Gross, W. (1920). Uber die Stellungsnahme auf abgelaufenen akuten psychose. *Zeitschrift fuer die Gesamte Neurologie Psychiatrie, 60*, 160-212.

McGlaschan, T. H. and Carpenter, W. T. Jr. (1976). An investigation of the post psychotic depressive syndrome. *American Journal of Psychiatry, 133*, 14-19.

McGlashan, T. H. and Johannessen, J. O. (1996). Early detection and intervention with schizophrenia: Rationale. *Schizophrenia Bulletin, 22*, 201-222.

McGlichrist, I. and Cutting, J. (1995). Somatic delusions in schizophrenia and the affective psychoses. *British Journal of Psychiatry, 167*, 350-361.

Meloy, J. (1984). Thought organization and primary process in the patients of schizophrenics. *British Journal of Medical Psychology, 57*, 279-281.

Meltzer, H. Y. and McGurk, S. R. (1999). The effects of clozapine, risperidone, and olanzapine on cognitive function in schizophrenia. *Schizophrenia Bulletin, 25*, 233-255.

Merriam, A. E., Kay, S., Opler, L. A., Kushner, S. F. and van Praag, H. M. (1990). Neurological signs and the positive-negative dimension in schizophrenia. *Biological Psychiatry, 28*, 181-192.

Merskey, H. (1965). The characteristics of persistent pain in psychological illness. *Journal of Psychosomatic Research, 9*, 291-298.

Meyer, E., Jacobsen, W., Edgerton, M. and Canter, A. (1960). Motivational patterns in patients seeking elective plastic surgery (women who seek rhinoplasty). *Psychosomatic Medicine, 22*, 193-199.

Milner, B. (1963). Effect of different brain lesions in card sorting. The role of the frontal lobes. *Archives of Neurology, 9*, 100-110.

Nuechterlein, K. H., Edell, W. S., Norris, M. and Dawson, M. E. (1986). Attentional vulnerability indicators, thought disorder, and negative symptoms. *Schizophrenia Bulletin, 12*, 408-426.

Oosthuizen, P., Lambert, T. and Castle, D. J. (1998). Dysmorphic concern: prevalence and associations with clinical variables. *Australia and New Zealand Journal of Psychiatry, 32*, 129-132.

Overall, J. E. and Gorham, D. R. (1962). Brief Psychiatric Rating Scale (BPRS). *Psychological Reports, 10*, 799-812.

Pantelis, C., Nelson, H. E. and Barnes, T. R. E. (1996). *Schizophrenia: A neuropsychological perspective*. Chichester, West Sussex: John Wiley and Sons.

Pattison, E. M. and Kahan, T. (1983). The deliberate self-harm syndrome. *American Journal of Psychiatry, 140*, 867-872.

Perry, W. and Braff, D. L. (1994). Information processing and thought disorder in schizophrenia. *American Journal of Psychiatry, 151*, 363-367.

Perry, W. and Braff, D. L. (1998). A multimethod approach to assessing perseveration in schizophrenia patients. *Schizophrenia Research, 33*, 69-77.

Perry, W., Geyer, M. A. and Braff, D. L. (1999). Sensorimotor gating and thought disturbance measured in close temporal proximity in schizophrenic patients. *Archives of General Psychiatry, 56*, 277-281.

Perry, W., Viglione, D. and Braff, D. L. (1992). The Ego Impairment Index and schizophrenia: a validation study. *Journal of Personality Assessment, 59*, 165-175.

Phillips, K. A. (1991). Body dysmorphic disorder: The distress of imagined ugliness. American *Journal of Psychiatry, 148*, 1138-1149.

Phillips, K. A. and McElroy, S. L. (1993). Insight, overvalued ideation, and delusional thinking in body dysmorphic disorder: Theoretical and treatment implications. *Journal of Nervous and Mental Disease, 181*, 699-702.

Phillips, K. A. and McElroy, S. L., Keck, P. E., Hudson, J. I. and Pope, H. G. Jr. (1994). A comparison of delusional and nondelusional body dysmorphic disorder in 100 cases. *Psychopharmacology Bulletin, 30*, 179-186.

Philips, C. and Hunter, M. (1982). Headache in a psychiatric population. *Journal of Nervous and Mental Disease, 170,* 34-40.

Pick, A. (1922). Stoerung der Orientierung am eigenen Koerper. *Psychologische Forschung, 1*, 303-315

Pickar, D. (1995). Prospects for pharmacotherapy of schizophrenia. *Lancet, 345(8949)*, 557-562.

Quinlan, D. M. and Harrow, M. (1974). Boundary disturbance in schizophrenia. *Journal of Abnormal Psychology, 83*, 533-541.

Rado, S. (1959). Dynamics and classification of disorder behavior. *American Journal of Psychiatry, 1*, 651-656.

Reitman, E. E. and Cleveland, S. E. (1964). Changes in body image following sensory deprivation in schizophrenic and control groups. *Journal of Abnormal and Social Psychology, 68*, 168-176.

Renik, O. D. and Fisher, S. (1968). Induction of body image boundary changes in male subjects. *Journal of Projective Techniques and Personality Assessment, 32*, 45-49.

Ritzler, B. and Rosenbaum, G. (1974). Proprioception in schizophrenics and normals: Effects of stimulus intensity and interstimulus interval. *Journal of Abnormal Psychology, 83*, 106-111.

Ritzler, B. (1977). Proprioception and schizophrenia: A replication study with nonschizophrenic patient controls. *Journal of Abnormal Psychology, 86*, 501-504.

Roehricht, F. and Priebe, S. (1996). Body image of patients with acute paranoid schizophrenia: A follow-up study. (Das Koerpererleben von Patienten mit einer akuten paranoiden Schizophrenie. Eine Verlaufsstudie.) *Nervenarzt, 67*, 602-607.

Roehricht, F. and Priebe, S. (1997). Disturbances of body experience in schizophrenic patients.(Stoerungen des Koerpererlebens bei schizophrenen Patienten.) *Fortschritte der Neurologie-Psychiatrie, 65*, 323-336.

Rosenbaum, G., Flenning, F. and Rosen, H. (1965). Effects of weight intensity on discrimination thresholds of normals and schizophrenics. *Journal of Abnormal Psychology,* 70, 446-450.

Rosenthal, S. H., Porter, K. A. and Coffey, B. (1990). Pain insensitivity in schizophrenia: Case report and review of the literature. *General Hospital Psychiatry, 12*, 319-322.

Roy, A., Thompson, R. and Kennedy, S. (1983). Depression in chronic schizophrenia. *British Journal of Psychiatry, 142*, 465-470.

Sacks, M. H., Carpenter, W. T. and Strauss, J. S. (1974). Recovery from delusions. *Archives of General Psychiatry, 30*, 117-120.

Saykin, J. A., Gur, R. C., Gur, R. E., Mozley, P. D., Mozley, L. H., Resnick, S. M, Kester, D. B. and Stafiniak, P. (1991). Neuropsychological function in schizophrenia: selective impairment in memory and learning. *Archives of General Psychiatry, 48*, 618-624.

Schafer, R. (1960). Bodies in Schizophrenic Rorschach Responses. *Journal of Projective Techniques, 24*, 267-281.

Schafer, R. (1986). *Projective Testing and Psychoanalysis. Selected Papers*. International Universities Press, INC.

Scheftel, S., Nathan, A. S., Razin, A. M. and Mezan, P. (1986). A case of radical facial self-mutilation: An unprecedented event and its impact. *Bulletin of the Menninger Clinic, 50*, 525-540.

Schilder, P. (1935). *The image and appearance of the human body*. London: Kegan Paul, Trench, Trubner and Co.

Schmoll, D. (1994). Coenaesthetische Schizophrenie. *Fortschritte der Neurologie Psychiatrie, 62*, 372-378.

Schmoll, D. and Koch, T. (1989). Leibgefuehlsstoerungen in der schizophrenen Psychose. Eine Kasuistik. *Nervenarzt, 60*, 619-627.

Schneider, F., Gur, R. C., Gur, R. E., Shtasel, D. L. (1995). Emotional processing in schizophrenia: Neurobehavioral probes in relation to psychopathology. *Schizophrenia Research, 17*, 67-75.

Schneider, K. (1959). *Klinische Psychopathologie, 12th ed.* Stuttgart: Georg Thieme Verlag, (5th eds. Translated by M. W. Hamilton. Clinical Psychopathology. New York: Grune and Stratton, 1976.)

Shore, D., Andreasen, D. J. and Cutler, N. R. (1978). Prediction of self-mutilation in hospitalized schizophrenics. *American Journal of Psychiatry 135*:1406-1407.

Schweitzer I. 1990 Genital self-amputation and the Klingsor Syndrome. *Australian and New Zealand Journal of Psychiatry, 24*, 566-569.

Silva, J. A., Leong, G. B. and Weinstock, R. (1989). A case of skin and ear self-mutilation. *Psychosomatics, 30*, 228-230.

Silverstein, M. L. and Zerwic, M. J. (1985). Clinical psychopathologic symptoms in neuropsychologically impaired and intact schizophrenics. *Journal of Consulting and Clinical Psychology, 53*, 267-268.

Siris, S. G. (1991). Diagnosis of secondary depression in schizophrenia: Implications for DSM-IV. *Schizophrenia Bulletin, 17*, 75-98.

Snaith, P. (1992). Body image disorders. *Psychotherapy and Psychosomatics, 58*, 119-124.

Sonneburn, C. K. and Vanstraelen, P. M. (1992). A retsospective study on self-inflicted burns. *General Hospital Psychiatry, 14*, 404-407.

Spear, F. G. (1967). Pain in psychiatric patients. *Journal of Psychosomatic Research, 11*,187-193.

SPSS. (1997). *SPSS Base 7.5 Application Guide*. Chicago, Illinois: SPSS.

Spohn, H. E. and Strauss, M. E. (1989). Relation of neuroleptic and anticholinergic medication to cognitive functions in schizophrenia. *Journal of Abnormal Psychology, 98*, 367-380.

Strauss, M. E. (1993). Relations of symptoms to cognitive deficits in schizophrenia. *Schizophrenia Bulletin, 19*, 215-231.

Strauss, S. (1989). Subjective experiences of schizophrenia: Toward a new dynamic psychiatry – II. *Schizophrenia Bulletin, 15*, 179-187.

Sugarman, A. A. and Cancro, R. (1964). Field dependence and sophistication of body concept in schizophrenics. *Journal of Nervous and Mental Disease, 138*, 119-123.

Sweeny, S. and Zamecnik, K. (1981). Predictors of self-mutilation in patients with schizophrenia. *American Journal of Psychiatry, 138*, 1086-1089.

Swensen, C. H. (1957). Empirical evaluations of human figure drawings. *Psychological Bulletin, 54*, 431-466.

Swensen, C. H. (1968). Empirical evaluations of human figure drawings: 1957-1966. *Psychological Bulletin, 70*, 20-44.

Taylor, M. A. and Abrams, R. (1984). Cognitive dysfunction in schizophrenia. *American Journal of Psychiatry, 141*, 196-201.

Taylor, P. J. (1995). Schizophrenia and the risk of violence. In S. R. Hirsh and D. R. Weinberger (Eds). *Schizophrenia*. Oxford: Blackwell Science Ltd.

Tollefson, G. D., Sanger, T. M., Lu, Y. and Thieme, M.E. (1998). Depressive signs and symptoms in schizophrenia: a prospective blinded trial of olanzapine and haloperidol. *Archives of General Psychiatry, 55*, 250-258.

Torrey, E. F. (1989). Headache in schizophrenia and seasonality of births. *Biological Psychiatry, 26*, 847-858.

Traub, A. C., Olson, R., Orbach, J. and Cardone, S. C. (1967). Psychophysical studies of body image: III. Initial studies of disturbance in a chronic schizophrenic group. *Archives of General Psychiatry, 17*, 664-670.

Twemlow, S. W., Gabbard, G.O. and Jones, F. C. (1982). The out-of-body experience: a phenomenological typology based on questionnaire responses. *American Journal of Psychiatry, 139*, 450-455.

Urist, J. (1977). The Rorschach test and the assessment of object relations. *Journal of Personality Assessment, 41*, 3-9.

Vanderkampt, H. (1970). Clinical anomalies in patients with schizophrenia. *Experimental Medicine and Surgery, 28*, 291-293.

Van Puttan, T. and May, P. R. A. (1978). 'Akinetic depression' in schizophrenia. *Archives of General Psychiatry, 35*, 1101-1107.

Varsamis, J., Adamson, J. D. (1976). Somatic symptoms in schizophrenia. *Canadian Psychiatric Association Journal, 21*, 1-6.

Vincent, K. R. and Harman, M. J. (1991). The Exner Rorschach: an analysis of its clinical validity. *Journal of Clinical Psychology, 47*, 596-599.

Wagner, E. E. and Frye, D. (1990). Diagnostic and intellectual implications of the fragmented Rorschach W:D ratio. *Perceptual and Motor Skills, 71*, 887-890.

Watkins, J. and Stauffacher, J. (1952). An index of pathological thinking in the Rorschach. *Journal of Projective Techniques, 16,* 276-286.

Watson, G. D., Chandarana, P. C. and Merskey, H. (1981). Relationships between pain and schizophrenia. *British Journal of Psychiatry, 138*, 33-36.

Weckowicz, T. E. and Sommer, R. (1960). Body image and self-concept in schizophrenia, an experimental study. *Journal of Mental Science, 106*, 17-39.

Weinberger, D. R., Berman, K. F. and Zec, R. F. (1986). Physiologic dysfunction of dorsolateral prefrontal cortex in schizophrenia: I. Regional cerebral blood flow evidence. *Archives of General Psychiatry, 4*, 114-124.

Weinberger, D. R., Torrey, E. F., Neophytides, A. N. and Wyatt, R.J. (1979). Lateral cerebral ventricular enlargement in chronic schizophrenia. *Archives of General Psychiatry, 36*, 735-739.

Weiser, M., Levy, A. and Neuman, M. (1993). Ear Stuffing: An unusual form of self-mutilation. *Journal of Nervous and Mental Disease, 181*, 587-588.

West, B. M. and Hecker, A.O. (1952). Peptic ulcer: Incidence and diagnosis in psychotic patients. *American Journal of Psychiatry, 109*, 35-37.

Young, D. A., Davila, R. and Scher, H. (1993). Unawareness of illness and neuropsychological performance in chronic schizophrenia. *Schizophrenia Research, 10*, 117-124.

Zung, W. W. K. (1965). A self-rating depression scale. *Archives of General Psychiatry, 12*, 63-70.

In: Adolescent Schizophrenia
Editors: J. T. Nillinghouse and R. P. Trotman
ISBN: 978-1-60692-370-2

Chapter VII

Sex Differences in Aggressive and Delinquent Behavior in Schizotypal Adolescents[1]

Amanda McMillan and Elaine Walker
Department of Psychology, Emory University, Atlanta, Georgia

There is a well-documented link between schizophrenia and antisocial behavior. For example, studies of violent offenders worldwide find a significantly elevated prevalence of schizophrenia and spectrum disorder diagnoses (Gosden, Kramp, Gabrielsen, and Sestoft, 2003; Arseneault, Moffitt, Caspi, Taylor, and Silva, 2000). Conversely, studies of patient populations reveal higher rates of antisocial behavior. In an investigation of a large Danish birth cohort in their forties, proportionately more of the men and women who developed schizophrenia were convicted of non-violent and violent crimes (Brennan, Mednick, and Hodgins, 2000). Similar results were obtained in investigations of population cohorts in Australia (Mullen, Burgess, Wallace, Palmer, and Ruschena, 2000), Israel (Stueve and Link, 1997), and New Zealand (Arseneault et al., 2000).

Investigations into the specific links between symptoms and antisocial behavior suggest that the severity of positive symptoms is the strongest predictor of aggressive and violent behavior. Further, some findings indicate that individuals at risk for developing schizophrenia and spectrum disorders are more likely to manifest antisocial behaviors. The link between premorbid antisocial behavior and psychosis has been examined in both retrospective and prospective longitudinal studies. In a retrospective study of childhood-onset schizophrenia, Schaeffer and Ross (2002) found a high proportion of parents reporting oppositional behavior, violence, aggression, temper tantrums, and rages as premorbid signs in their children. Similarly, Arsenault et al. (2000) found that individuals with schizophrenia-spectrum disorders were more likely to have a childhood history of conduct disorder.

[1] This research was supported by Grant # RO1 MH62066-01 awarded to Dr. Walker from the National Institute of Mental Health.

The rate of premorbid antisocial behaviors appears to increase with age as the individual approaches late adolescence/early adulthood, the peak risk period for the onset of psychosis. In examining the premorbid developmental course through childhood, Neumann, Grimes, Walker and Baum (1995), used the Child Behavior Checklist (CBCL) and found a significant increase in aggressive behaviors in preschizophrenic children between 8 and 12 years of age. Two empirically-derived clusters were observed; Cluster I manifested early onset and escalating behavioral abnormalities, whereas Cluster II did not begin to differ from controls until adolescence. By 8 to 12 years, Cluster I was not only exhibiting more aggressive behavior than control subjects but Cluster II individuals as well. Using a similar retrospective design, Rossi, Pollice, Daneluzzo, Marinangeli and Stratta (2000) collected maternal reports of behavioral abnormalities for five age periods from birth through adolescence and found that all behavioral abnormality dimensions, including delinquent and aggressive behavior, were higher in the patient group when compared to the normal controls, and increased consistently with age.

Prospective studies of children at high risk for psychotic disorders yield similar findings. Bearden et al. (2000) followed a population cohort from childhood into adulthood to identify behavioral problems that preceded schizophrenia. They assessed a range of behaviors, including emotional reactivity and hostility, when the subjects were aged 4 and 7 years. Their findings indicate that a progression from initial social deficits to more severe behavioral deviance precedes adult-onset schizophrenia. Bergman, Wolfson and Walker (1997) examined behavioral problems in the offspring (mean age 9.75 years) of parents with a diagnosis of schizophrenia. Compared to those whose parents had no mental illness, the high-risk children exhibited elevated levels of externalizing behaviors (aggression and delinquency) on the CBCL. Further, the rate of behavior problems increased from the initial assessment to the follow-up, one year later. In a subsequent report from the Edinburgh High Risk Study, Miller, Byrne, Hodges, Lawrie and Johnstone (2002) obtained reports on the CBCL at two time periods, prior to age 13 and from ages 13-16. The high-risk individuals who later developed schizophrenia displayed significantly more externalizing behaviors when compared to those who did not go on to develop the illness. Specifically, prior to age 13, high risk children who later developed schizophrenia were more aggressive, and the difference became stronger in the 13-16 age period, with a much higher incidence of aggressive and delinquent behaviors in those individuals who later developed schizophrenia.

There is evidence that premorbid externalizing behaviors are linked with more pronounced cognitive impairment and clinical symptoms in patients. Baum and Walker (1995) used retrospective CBCL data, and found that patients who showed more childhood aggression and delinquency between ages 8 and16 years also manifested greater cognitive disorganization in adulthood. Neumann, Baum, Walker and Lewine (1996) found that escalating childhood delinquency predicted deficits in adult motor functioning, whereas both childhood delinquency and aggression predicted cognitive impairment. Replicating this pattern of findings, in a study of adult-onset schizophrenia patients, the presence of premorbid disciplinary problems was associated with more pronounced adult neuropsychological deficits (Silverstein, Mavrolefteros, and Turnbull, 2003). Among the various disciplinary problems, physical violence showed the strongest relation with adult neuropsychological deficits. Additionally, there is evidence to suggest that the association between childhood behavior and adult cognitive function may reflect underlying brain dysfunction. Walker, Lewine and Neumann (1996) found that premorbid externalizing problems in childhood were related with greater brain abnormalities in adult schizophrenia patients. Specifically, increases in delinquent behaviors were associated with ventricular enlargement and smaller whole brain volume.

Schizotypal Personality and Antisocial Behavior

Schizotypal personality disorder (SPD) is a syndrome that involves deficits in interpersonal functioning, and perceptual and ideational abnormalities. There is an extensive body of literature showing that schizotypal signs are more prevalent in the biological relatives of patients with schizophrenia and other psychotic disorders. This has led to the assumption that there is a genetic link between schizophrenia and SPD. Further, schizotypal signs often predate the onset of schizophrenia, so the manifestation appears to represent a prodromal developmental phase of the disorder in some patients.

As is the case with schizophrenia, there is evidence that SPD is associated with an increase in antisocial behavior. A study of schizotypal symptoms and interpersonal behaviors in undergraduate students revealed that students who scored higher on measures of perceptual aberration and magical ideation were more likely to engage in hostile interactions, including expressions of irritation, belligerence and anger (Shean and Wais, 2000). Similarly, in a study aimed at differentiating between positive and negative schizotypy in an undergraduate population, those with more positive symptoms (perceptual distortions) also scored higher on measures of antisocial personality disorder (Dinn, Harris, Acyicegi, Greene, and Andover, 2002). Raine, Venables, Mednick and Mellingen (2002) looked at persistently schizotypal adults and found that they scored higher on measures of conduct disorder, including both physical and verbal aggression, than controls. In a retrospective study of adolescents with SPD, Walker, Baum and Diforio (1998) obtained parental reports of behavior problems throughout childhood. When compared to normal subjects, there was a significant developmental increase in externalizing behaviors in the schizotypal adolescents, especially in the early adolescent age period (12-15 years). In summary, research utilizing a variety of methodologies has revealed that schizophrenia-spectrum disorders are associated with an increase in the rate of antisocial behavior, ranging from interpersonal hostility to physical aggression to violence. Further, it appears that there is a developmental increase in the risk for these behaviors, with a marked rise in adolescence.

There is also evidence that gender moderates the relation between antisocial behavior and schizophrenia spectrum disorders. In a review of the literature, Walker, Walder, Lewine and Loewy (2002) found that, with increasing age, preschizophrenic males are characterized as exhibiting increased externalizing behaviors while females show a higher rate of internalizing behaviors. Summarizing the findings on violence and schizophrenia, Hodgins, Hiscoke and Freese (2003) conclude that, as is the case in the general population, the presence of violent behaviors prior to the onset of schizophrenia is much more common among men than women. But, along with other investigators, they also note evidence that schizophrenia more significantly increases the risk for violence in women than in men

(Brennan et al., 2000; Hodgins and Janson, 2002). In other words, the presence of a schizophrenia-spectrum disorder raises the risk for antisocial behavior to a greater extent in women. Further, in the controlled environment of an inpatient ward, women with psychotic disorders are just as likely to behave violently as are their male counterparts (Newhill, Mulvey, and Lidz, 1995).

The Emory University Adolescent Development Project: A Prospective Study of Schizotypal Adolescents

We have explored the relation between schizotypal symptoms and antisocial behavior in the Emory University Adolescent Development Project. Based on past findings, it was predicted that adolescents who meet diagnostic criteria for SPD will manifest a higher rate of externalizing behavior problems, including delinquency and aggression, than adolescents with no Axis II disorder. It was also predicted that ratings of the positive schizotypal symptoms, but not negative symptoms, will be significantly linked with delinquent and aggressive behavior. Finally, we examined the effect of sex on the nature and strength of the relation between antisocial behavior and schizotypy.

Currently enrolled participants in the Emory Study are 118 children, ranging in age from 12 to 18 years. Children with personality disorders were recruited through an announcement directed at parents of youth with adjustment problems. The announcement described the key diagnostic criteria for schizotypal personality disorder in lay terms. Telephone screening interviews were conducted, and prospective participants who seemed likely to meet criteria for SPD, or another personality disorder, were scheduled for the research assessment. Healthy participants were primarily recruited through a University based registry of children in the Atlanta area. Demographic characteristics of the sample are presented in Table 1. Exclusion criteria were neurological disorder, mental retardation, Axis I disorder, and substance abuse/addiction.

A battery of diagnostic measures was administered, including the Structured Interview for DSM-IV Personality disorders (SIDP-IV) (Pfohl, Blum, and Zimmerman, 1997) and the Structured Clinical Interview for Axis I DSM-IV Disorders (SCID) (First, Spitzer, Gibbon, and Williams, 1995). Interviews were administered by trained graduate-level examiners, and diagnoses were made by review of the videotaped interviews and other materials by research project staff, including a licensed psychologist and psychiatrist. As expected, the announcement elicited responses from parents whose children manifested a range of problems, and met criteria for SPD as well as other Axis II disorders. Consistent with previous reports, the rate of comorbid personality disorder was 51%.

Parents of the children completed the Child Behavior Checklist. This behavioral rating Scale contains 104 items (CBCL; Achenbach, 1991; Achenbach and Edelbrock, 1981). The CBCL was chosen because it contains items that measure a broad range of behavioral problems and yields scores for seven behavior problem dimensions, including two that index externalized behavior problems and are the focus of the present study, namely "delinquent behavior," and "aggressive behavior." As described above, previous studies have shown that scores on these scales predict subsequent diagnosis with SPD and schizophrenia. Also, the CBCL has been demonstrated to have good reliability. For example, in a study of parents' reports of normal and disturbed children (aged 4–16 years), the interclass correlations were .90 or greater for interparent agreement, 1-week test–retest reliability, and inter-interviewer reliability (Achenbach and Edelbrock, 1981). Composite scores for the CBCL behavior problem dimensions are derived by summing the items in the particular behavior dimension. The mother served as the informant about childhood behavior for most of the participants.

Table 1. Subject Demographic Information and Medication Status

	SPD (n=32)	OPD (n=37)	NoPD (n=49)
Age			
Mean	14.25	14.34	14.08
Standard Deviation	1.723	1.697	1.935
Sex			
Males	21	19	27
Females	11	18	22
PD Comorbidity (%)	72	32	0
Medication Status			
Stimulant	8	1	3
Antidepressant	5	3	3
Both	3	4	2

Results of Data Analyses

Diagnostic group comparisons revealed no significant difference in mean age, however, the SPD group included a higher proportion of males than the other groups, $\chi^2 = 4.90$, p=.03.

An ANOVA was conducted on the CBCL externalizing behavior ratings, with diagnostic group and sex as the independent variables. Figure 1 displays the aggression scores by sex and diagnostic group. The analysis of aggression scores revealed a significant main effect for diagnostic group, $F(2,110) = 4.82$, $p<.01$, and a significant Diagnostic group X Sex interaction $F(2,110) = 3.08$, $p<.05$. T-test comparisons showed that the diagnostic group differences in aggression ratings for males did not reach statistical significance. But among females, the normal controls had significantly lower scores for aggression than the SPD, $t(36) = 3.10$, $p<.01$, and other personality disorder (OPD), $t(36) = 2.88$, $p<.01$, groups. Consistent with past reports, among normals, males showed significantly more aggression than females, $t(45) = 2.35$, $p<.05$. In contrast, there were no sex differences in ratings for aggression in the SPD or OPD groups. This is counter to some past reports which indicated that antisocial behavior is greater in preschizophrenic males.

The analysis of delinquency scores revealed a significant main effect for diagnostic group, $F(2,110) = 7.07$, $p<.001$, but the interaction did not reach significance. Figure 2 displays the delinquency scores by sex and diagnostic group. T-test comparisons showed that there was a significant group difference in delinquency, with the OPD group showing a higher mean score than the normal group, $t(74)= 3.59$, $p<.001$, and the SPD group $t(74)= 2.19$, $p<.05$. This is consistent with the fact that the OPD group contained a subgroup with antisocial personality/conduct disorder. The differences between the normal and SPD group approached significance, $t(74)= 1.62$, $p<.10$, with the SPD group showing more delinquency. Among normals, consistent with past reports, males showed a trend toward more delinquency than females, $t(45)= 1.64$, $p<.10$. There were no sex differences in ratings for delinquency in the SPD or OPD groups.

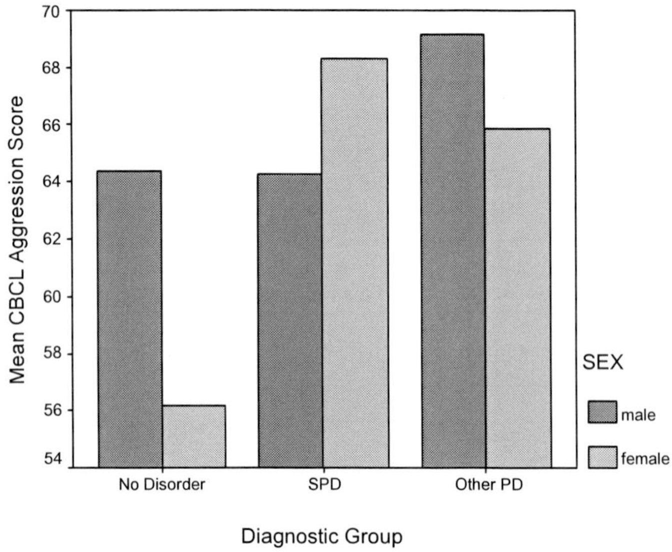

Figure 1. Mean aggression score by diagnostic group

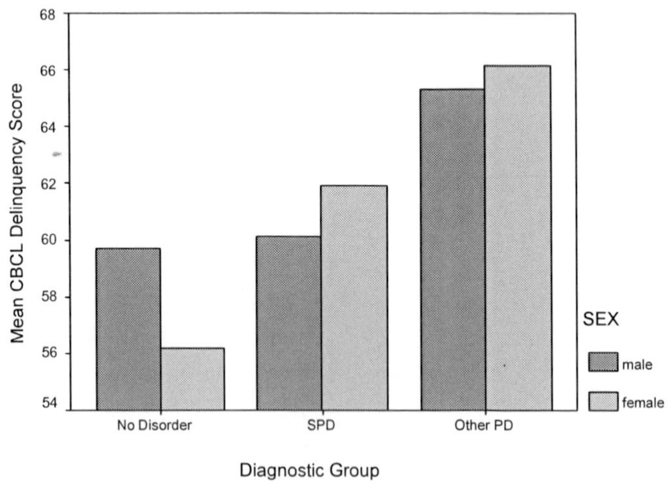

Figure 2. Mean delinquency score by diagnostic group

Correlational analyses were conducted to examine the relation of SPD symptoms with delinquent and aggressive behavior. Given the significant sex differences in the behavioral profiles of the diagnostic groups, analyses were conducted separately by sex. The results are listed in Table 2, for the three diagnostic groups combined. (Analyses were conducted with the combined groups because the separate diagnostic groupings are based on the symptom ratings.) As shown, for boys there were no significant relations between ratings of SPD symptoms and delinquent and aggressive behavior. In contrast, for girls, there were significant positive associations between aggression and almost all of the SPD symptoms: ideas of reference, odd beliefs/magical thinking, unusual perceptual experiences, odd thinking and speech, suspiciousness, inappropriate or constricted affect, and odd behavior or appearance. The only symptoms that were not associated with increased aggression were lack of friends and social anxiety. Thus for girls, but not boys, more severe positive schizotypal symptom ratings were associated with higher parent-rated aggression in the child. The only significant relation for delinquency was with ratings of suspiciousness in females.

As described, the sex differences revealed in our group comparisons ran counter to our predictions based on past reports. We therefore sought to determine whether psychotropic medication might be contributing to these effects. Specifically, a substantial number of the research participants, especially those meeting diagnostic criteria for SPD, were currently taking psychotropic medication. The most common were stimulant and antidepressant medication. For the total sample, 44% had a lifetime history of psychotropic medication, 33% were currently on medication, and 23% were receiving, or had received, two or more medications simultaneously. The classes of psychotropics and the number of participants taking each are listed in Table 1. For about one half of those on medication, the prescribing physician was a pediatrician. The breakdown for current medication was as follows: Antidepressant alone n=11; Stimulant alone n=12; Antipsychotic alone n=2; Antidepressant and Antipsychotic n=5; Antidepressant and Stimulant n=9; Antipsychotic and Stimulant n=1; All three medications n=4.

We first sought to determine whether medication status was linked with the behavior ratings. Regression analysis was conducted using current status on the three classes of psychotropics (stimulants, antidepressants and antipsychotics) as the predictor variables, and ratings on the aggression and delinquency factors as the dependent variables. The results showed that, taken together, the medication variables accounted for a significant proportion of the variance in aggression ratings, $F(3,112)= 4.93$, $p<.01$. As independent predictors, both stimulant and antidepressant use showed a trend toward significant association with higher aggression ratings. When the same analysis was conducted on the delinquency rating, the equation did not reach significance, $F(3,112)= 1.74$, $p=.13$. But, stimulant use was a significant independent predictor, $t=2.14$, $p<.05$. Again, medication was linked with higher ratings.

Table 2. Correlations (Pearson) between ratings of schizotypal symptoms and delinquent and aggressive behavior by sex

	Schizotypal Symptoms									
	Ideas of Reference	Magical Thinking	Perceptual Experiences	Odd Thinking	Paranoid Ideation	Inappropriate Affect	Odd Behavior	Lack of Friends	Social Anxiety	Total Symptoms
Males n=67										
Delinquency	-0.032	0.031	-0.152	-0.178	0.128	-0.013	-0.051	0.032	-0.058	-0.042
Aggression	-0.043	0.110	0.001	-0.119	0.035	0.107	-0.002	0.086	-0.089	0.027
Females n=51										
Delinquency	0.124	0.180	-0.024	0.158	0.287*	0.113	0.190	0.089	-0.020	0.183
Aggression	0.257	0.332**	0.247*	0.393**	0.263*	0.288*	0.471**	0.177	0.149	0.395**

n=66 for males in the Paranoid Ideation Symptom rating
* Correlation is significant at the 0.05 level (1-tailed)
** Correlation is significant at the 0.01 level (1-tailed)

When the diagnostic group X sex ANOVA of delinquency scores was conducted, excluding those on stimulants or antidepressants, the results were similar to those obtained with the entire sample. There was a significant main effect for diagnostic group, $F(2,79)= 8.75$, $p<.001$, but the interaction did not reach significance. T-test comparisons showed that there was a significant group difference in delinquency, with the OPD group showing a higher mean score than the normal group, $t(60)= 3.92$, $p<.01$, and the SPD group, $t(44)= 2.38$, $p<.02$. There was a trend toward higher delinquency ratings in the SPD group compared to the normal control subjects, $t(60)= 1.37$, $p<.10$. Consistent with past reports among normals, males showed a trend toward more delinquency than females, $t=2.12$, $p= .06$. There were no sex differences in ratings for delinquency in the SPD or OPD groups.

When the Diagnostic group X Sex ANOVA was conducted on the aggression scores, excluding those on antidepressants or stimulants, the results differed from those reported above. There was a significant main effect for diagnostic group, $F(2,90)= 4.91$, $p<.01$, but the sex X diagnostic group interaction did not reach significance. The OPD group scored higher on aggression than the normal gro.up, $t(60)= 3.00$, $p<.01$. The SPD adolescents showed more aggression than the normal control group, $t(60)= 1.85$, $p<.05$. There was no difference between the SPD and OPD groups.

The change in the findings for aggression ratings that resulted from the exclusion of those on medication appears to be a consequence of the differential effect of medication on externalizing behavior in males and females. Figure 3 displays the aggression scores, by medication status (stimulant or antidepressant), sex and diagnostic group.

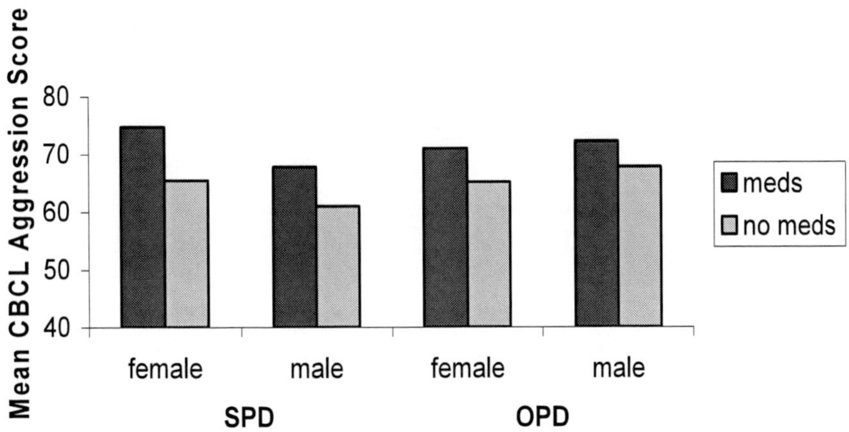

Figure 3. Mean aggression score by diagnostic group, gender and medication status

As illustrated in Figure 3, both males and females on medication score higher on aggression than those not on medication. We tested the relation of medication status with behavior ratings for males within diagnostic group. For normal control and SPD males, those on medication scored significantly higher on aggression than those off medication, $t(23)= 4.18$, $p<05$, and $t(23)= 2.06$, $p<05$. As shown, the number of female subjects in some groups was too small to permit statistical tests. We therefore combined the two personality disorder groups to test for the medication effect in females. In the combined SPD/OPD group, both females and males currently on medication had significantly higher aggression ratings than their same-sex counterparts, $t(27)= 1.87$, $p<05$, $t(38)= 1.71$, $p<05$, respectively.

Discussion

Consistent with previous reports, we find elevations in aggressive and delinquent behavior in adolescents with SPD. But the pattern differed by sex, and appeared to be influenced by medication status. These findings suggest that the association between SPD and antisocial behavior is complex.

Our analyses revealed that aggression ratings were elevated in participants who were receiving antidepressant or stimulant medication. When the participants who were on these drugs were excluded, the analyses revealed a pattern of diagnostic group differences in aggression and delinquency that did not vary by sex. Namely, the SPD adolescents manifested more aggression and a trend toward more delinquency than the healthy adolescents. These findings converge with past studies that have found a link between SPD and elevations in antisocial behaviors.

It is important to note that although the CBCL aggression and delinquency dimensions include items that pertain to criminal activity and physical aggression, adolescents can score high on these scales because they manifest noncriminal delinquent activity (e.g., noncompliance with adult authority figures) and verbal aggression. Thus the antisocial behaviors manifested by these SPD adolescents do not necessarily include the violent or criminal behaviors that have been the subject of much of the research on schizophrenia and antisocial behavior.

The findings of the present investigation diverge from past reports with respect to sex differences. Past research on schizophrenia has typically shown that male patients manifest more aggressive and criminal behavior than females (Steinert, Wiebe, and Gebhardt, 1999). Similarly, studies of the childhood precursors of schizophrenia-spectrum disorders have consistently revealed more aggressive and delinquent behavior in preschizophrenic males. We do not find this sex difference in the present study; among SPD youth, males and females displayed comparable levels of antisocial behavior.

There are several possible explanations for the discrepancy between the present results and those of previous investigations. First, it may be that the sex difference in premorbid antisocial behavior does not extend into the adolescent period, after the onset of the SPD syndrome. In other words, once the severity of schizotypal signs exceeds the threshold for SPD criteria, females may show a more dramatic developmental rise in antisocial behavior. This could, therefore, eliminate the premorbid sex difference. Such an interpretation is consistent with the notion that schizophrenia-spectrum disorders are linked with a more dramatic increase in antisocial behavior in females than in males.

Alternatively, the present findings may indicate a cohort shift in the rate of antisocial behavior among females. Thus, the previously reported sex difference in antisocial behavior among those with spectrum disorders may not hold for current cohorts. One trend that could produce cohort changes is the increase in the administration of psychotropics, especially antidepressants and stimulants, to youth. This increase has been documented over the past two decades, and is especially pronounced in the United States. It has been shown that these two medications are being prescribed, often by pediatricians, to children who manifest a variety of adjustment problems. It is therefore not surprising that many of the youth in our samples who meet diagnostic criteria for Axis II disorders have taken psychotropic medications.

There is suggestive evidence that these medications increase some externalizing behaviors in children. Barkley (1977) in a review analysis of relevant clinical trials reported increased irritability in children receiving stimulant medications. This medication-induced agitation could contribute to increases in aggression and delinquency. Recent reviews also cite irritability as an adverse side effect to stimulant usage (Greenhill, 2001)I®Additionally, Mann and Kapur (1991) cite reports of multiple and pharmacologically diverse antidepressants associated with the appearance of suicidal and aggressive behavior. Specifically, the SSRI fluvoxamine has been indicated for triggering aggression and violence, particularly in children and adolescents (Breggin, 2001). Vitiello and Swedo (2004) report increased agitation, particularly in children receiving SSRIs when compared to those receiving a placebo. Of course, it may also be that elevations in antisocial behaviors precede and/or precipitate the administration of medication. In future studies, we will explore this question by examining the relation between developmental changes in behavior and changes in medication status.

Our hypothesis, that antisocial behaviors would be linked with more pronounced positive schizotypal symptoms, received partial support. In this sample, the relation was only observed among females. Specifically, females with higher ratings on positive symptoms were also rated by their parents as showing greater aggressive behavior. This may parallel the findings on sex differences in violence in adult schizophrenia patients. Again, the link between antisocial tendencies and schizophrenia-spectrum signs may be stronger in females. In summary, the present findings lend further support to the notion that SPD, like schizophrenia, is associated with higher rates of antisocial behavior.

Finally, the relationship between antisocial behavior and vulnerability to schizophrenia may provide yet another opportunity for early identification and intervention. Interestingly, an environmental enrichment program aimed at reducing both schizotypal personality and antisocial behavior produced a lower incidence of schizotypal and criminal outcomes in participants, suggesting a possible interaction between the two distinct sets of problematic behaviors (Raine, Mellingen, Liu, Venables, and Mednick, 2003).

References

Achenbach, T. (1991). *Child Behavior Checklist.* Department of Psychiatry, University of Vermont, Burlington, VT.

Achenbach, T., and Edelbrock, C. (1981). Behavioral problems and competencies reported by parents of normal and disturbed children aged four through sixteen. *Monographs of the Society for Research in Child Development, 46*(1), 82.

Arseneault, L., Moffitt, T., Caspi, A., Taylor, P., and Silva, P. (2000). Mental disorders and violence in a total birth cohort: Results from the Dunedin study. *Archives of General Psychiatry, 57*(10), 979-986.

Barkley, R. (1977). A review of stimulant drug research with hyperactive children. *Journal of Child Psychology and Psychiatry, 18*, 137-165.

Baum, K., and Walker, E. (1995). Childhood behavioral precursors of adult symptom dimensions in schizophrenia. *Schizophrenia Research, 16*, 111-120.

Bearden, C., Rosso, I., Hollister, J., Sanchez, L., Hadley, T., and Cannon, T. (2000). A prospective cohort study of childhood behavioral deviance and language abnormalities as predictors of adult schizophrenia. *Schizophrenia Bulletin, 26*(2), 395-410.

Bergman, A., Wolfson, M., and Walker, E. (1997). Neuromotor functioning and behavior problems in children at risk for psychopathology. *Journal of Abnormal Child Psychology, 25*(3), 229-237.

Breggin, P. (2001). Fluvoxamine as a cause of stimulation, mania and aggression with a critical analysis of the FDA-approved label. *International Journal of Risk and Safety in Medicine, 14*, 71-86.

Brennan, P., Mednick, S., and Hodgins, S. (2000). Major mental disorders and criminal violence in a Danish birth cohort. *Archives of General Psychiatry, 57*(5), 494-500.

Dinn, W., Harris, C., Acyicegi, A., Greene, P., and Andover, M. (2002). Positive and negative schizotypy in a student sample: Neurocognitive and clinical correlates. *Schizophrenia Research, 56*, 171-185.

First, M., Spitzer, R., Gibbon, M., and Williams, J. (1995). *Structured Clinical Interview for the DSM-IV Axis I Disorders* (SCID-I), Patient Edition. American Psychiatric Press, Washington, DC.

Gosden, N., Kramp, P., Gabrielsen, G., and Sestoft, D. (2003). Prevalence of mental disorders among 15-17 year-old male adolescent remand prisoners in Denmark. *Acta Psychiatrica Scandinavica, 107*, 102-110.

Greenhill, L. (2001). Clinical effects of stimulant medication in ADHD. In M. Solanto and A. Arnsten (Eds.), *Stimulant drugs and ADHD: Basic and clinical neuroscience* (Vol. xii, pp. 31-71). London: Oxford University Press.

Hodgins, S., Hiscoke, U., and Freese, R. (2003). The antecedents of aggressive behavior among men with schizophrenia: A prospective investigation of patients in community treatment. *Behavioral Sciences and the Law, 21*, 523-546.

Hodgins, S., and Janson, C. (2002). *Criminality and violence among the mentally disordered: The Stockholm Project Metropolitan* (Vol. xi). New York: Cambridge University Press.

Mann, J., and Kapur, S. (1991). The emergence of suicidal ideation and behavior during antidepressant pharmacology. *Archives of General Psychiatry, 48*(11), 1027-1033.

Miller, P., Byrne, M., Hodges, A., Lawrie, S., and Johnstone, E. (2002). Childhood behaviour, psychotic symptoms and psychosis onset in young people at high risk of schizophrenia: early findings from the Edinburgh High Risk Study. *Psychological Medicine, 32*, 173-179.

Mullen, P., Burgess, P., Wallace, C., Palmer, S., and Ruschena, D. (2000). Community care and criminal offending in schizophrenia. *Lancet, 355*(9204), 614-617.

Neumann, C., Baum, K., Walker, E., and Lewine, R. (1996). Childhood behavioral precursors of adult neuropsychological functioning in schizophrenia. *Neuropsychiatry, Neuropsychology, and Behavioral Neurology, 9*(4), 221-229.

Neumann, C., Grimes, K., Walker, E., and Baum, K. (1995). Developmental Pathways to Schizophrenia: Behavioral Subtypes. *Journal of Abnormal Psychology, 104*(4), 558-566.

Newhill, C., Mulvey, E., and Lidz, C. (1995). Characteristics of violence in the community by female patients seen in a psychiatric emergency service. *Psychiatric Services, 46*(8), 785-789.

Pfohl, B., Blum, N., and Zimmerman, M. (1997). *Structured Interview for DSM-IV Personality* (SIDP-IV). American Psychiatric Press, Washington, DC.

Raine, A., Mellingen, K., Liu, J., Venables, P., and Mednick, S. (2003). Effects of environmental enrichment at ages 3-5 years on schizotypal personality and antisocial behavior at ages 17 and 23 years. *The American Journal of Psychiatry, 160*(9), 1627-1635.

Raine, A., Venables, P., Mednick, S., and Mellingen, K. (2002). Increased psychophysiological arousal and orienting at ages 3 and 11 years in persistently schizotypal adults. *Schizophrenia Research, 54*, 77-85.

Rossi, A., Pollice, R., Daneluzzo, E., Marinangeli, M., and Stratta, P. (2000). Behavioral neurodevelopment abnormalities and schizophrenic disorder: A retrospective evaluation with the Childhood Behavior Checklist (CBCL). *Schizophrenia Research, 44*, 121-128.

Schaeffer, J., and Ross, R. (2002). Childhood-onset schizophrenia: Premorbid and prodromal diagnostic and treatment histories. *Journal of the American Academy of Childhood and Adolescent Psychiatry, 41*(5), 538-545.

Shean, G., and Wais, A. (2000). Interpersonal behavior and schizotypy. *The Journal of Nervous and Mental Diseases, 188*(12), 842-846.

Silverstein, M., Mavrolefteros, G., and Turnbull, A. (2003). Premorbid factors in relation to motor, memory, and executive functions deficits in adult schizophrenia. *Schizophrenia Research, 61*, 271-280.

Steinert, T., Wiebe, C., and Gebhardt, R. (1999). Aggressive behavior against self and others among first-admission patients with schizophrenia. *Psychiatric Services, 50*(1), 85-90.

Stueve, A., and Link, B. (1997). Violence and psychiatric disorders: Results from an epidemiological study of young adults in Israel. *Psychiatric Quarterly, 68*(4), 327-342.

Vitiello, B., and Swedo, S. (2004). Antidepressant medications in children. *The New England Journal of Medicine, 350*(15), 1489-1491.

Walker, E., Baum, K., and Diforio, D. (1998). Developmental changes in the behavioral expression of vulnerability for schizophrenia. In M. Lenzenweger and R. Dworkin (Eds.), *Origins and development of schizophrenia: Advances in experimental psychopathology* (pp. 469-491). Washington, DC: American Psychological Association.

Walker, E., Lewine, R., and Neumann, C. (1996). Childhood behavioral characteristics and adult brain morphology in schizophrenia. *Schizophrenia Research, 22*, 93-101.

Walker, E., Walder, D., Lewine, R., and Loewy, R. (2002). Sex differences in the origins and premorbid development of schizophrenia. In F. Lewis-Hall and T. Williams (Eds.), *Psychiatric illness in women: Emerging treatments and research* (Vol. xxii, pp. 193-214). Washington, DC: American Psychiatric Publishing, Inc.

In: Adolescent Schizophrenia
Editors: J. T. Nillinghouse and R. P. Trotman

ISBN: 978-1-60692-370-2

Chapter VIII

Fetal Origins of Antisocial Personality Disorder and Schizophrenia: Evidence from the Dutch Hunger Winter

Richard Neugebauer[1, 2, 3, 4] ***and Ezra Susser***[1,5]

[1]Epidemiology of Developmental Brain Disorders Department, New York State Psychiatric Institute, New York, NY [2]G.H. Sergievsky Center, Columbia University, New York, NY, US

[3] International Program on Refugee Trauma, New York, N.Y., US

[4]The Department of International Health and Development, School of Public Health and Tropical Medicine, Tulane University [5] Department of Epidemiology, Mailman School of Public Health, Columbia University, New York, N.Y., US

INTRODUCTION

Risk factors for mortality and morbidity are divisible into three categories: those present before conception, others occurring postpartum and finally, those that operate in the interval between conception and birth. Until comparatively recently, this last period received limited attention in epidemiological research on psychiatric and (to a lesser degree) other disorders first emerging beyond the childhood years. One notable exception is the early and sustained interest in possible prenatal viral etiology of schizophrenia. Nonetheless, the operation of genetic factors, present at conception, and of macro and micro-level environmental factors, in the postnatal period were the primary focus of attention.

The past two decades have witnessed a growing interest in the prenatal and perinatal origins of adolescent and adult onset somatic and psychiatric diseases. Early, ground breaking work by Ravelli in the 1970s on prenatal nutrition and adult onset obesity (Ravelli et al., 1976) was followed two decades later by studies on low birth weight and raised risk for cardiovascular disease (Barker, 2003a; Barker, 2003b; Roseboom et al., 2001; Leon,

2001; Harding, 2001) A separate vein of research, emerging in the 1980s, examined prenatal and perinatal factors in risk for psychiatric disorders, initially motivated by an interest in a 'neurodevelopmental hypothesis' of schizophrenaia (Cannon, Kendell, Susser and Jones, 2003), now broadened to include a life course approach to neuropsychiatric disorders (Terry and Susser, 2001). These two research initiatives link the knowledge of established perinatal risk factors for diseases of early life, acquired through several decades of pediatric and perinatal epidemiologic research, with an equally extensive literature on the distribution and determinants of adult onset disorders, thereby creating conditions for a greatly enhanced understanding of both the proximal and distal etiologies of disease and dysfunction across the life span. Some initial scientific insights yielded by this approach in the area of psychiatric disorders, specifically, of ASPD (ASPD) and schizophrenia, are the subject of the present chapter.

HISTORICAL DISASTER, EPIDEMIOLOGICAL OPPORTUNITY:DUTCH HUNGER WINTER 1944-1945

In October 1944, the German army blockaded food supplies to the Western Netherlands as punishment for Dutch involvement in the planned Allied invasion of Europe. Before the October blockade, the food supply had been adequate; in May 1945, following the German retreat, it became plentiful again. In the intervening months, however, the Dutch population, particularly in the larger cities, received increasingly meager food rations, a circumstance that was rendered even more difficult by an especially harsh winter (Burger, Drummond, and Sandstead, 1947). Hence, Dutch women who were pregnant in October 1944, and others who conceived in the following months, experienced declining food supplies at varying points in gestation.

This wartime catastrophe, occurring in a previously well nourished industrialized nation, created a strategic epidemiological opportunity to examine the association of prenatal nutritional deficiency of varying intensity imposed at different points in intrauterine development with postnatal health and cognitive outcomes. Zena Stein and Mervyn Susser were the first researchers to appreciate the potential of this historical disaster to yield a rich harvest of epidemiological good. The fundamental design of the present analyses is based upon the initial work of these investigators, Famine and Human Development (Stein et al., 1975). While the work of Stein and Susser focused on the impact of prenatal malnutrition on measured intelligence of male offspring at age 18, the historical conditions created by the Dutch Famine continue to offer a unique research opportunity for evaluating the increasingly longer term effects of this complex prenatal exposure on health and disease at each stage of the advancing life cycle of the exposed individuals.

The findings reported in this chapter link in utero famine exposure to ASPD and schizophrenia, thereby providing important evidence of a possible association between prenatal nutrition, brain development and subsequent postnatal psychopathology. The sections on each disorder begin with a brief account of findings from other investigations adopting a neurodevelopmental perspective, followed by a detailed account of our study methods, analysis, findings and conclusions. With each set of findings, we include an essential examination of alternative explanations and study limitations.

ANTISOCIAL PERSONALITY DISORDER

BACKGROUND

The causes of antisocial behavior, of ASPD and of its developmental precursor, conduct disorder, have received macro-level research attention for many decades. Striking regional differences and rapid secular variations in rates of violent crime argue persuasively for the profound influence of social, economic and community forces on antisocial behavior (Olds et al., 1998; Sampson, Raudenbush and Earls,1997). Nonetheless, biological, especially micro-level environmental, risk factors for antisocial behavior, including prenatal and perinatal factors, have garnered increasing scientific, public health, and policy interest, (Reiss, and Roth., 1993) especially when such factors may be amenable to intervention.

Most research in this field on humans (as contrasted with animal models) has necessarily been confined to observational studies. Numerous case control investigations have examined whether perinatal or obstetric complications occur more frequently among persons with a criminal record as compared with non-criminals (Raine, 1993). Prospective studies have tested whether the offspring of women with prenatal or obstetric complications have an increased risk for violent criminal offending as compared with offspring of women with comparatively unremarkable pregnancies. The authors of one study (Raine et al., 1994) found that such complications conferred risk only when conditioned on maternal rejection in the first postnatal year.

Despite the design strengths of these studies, especially of the cohort studies, research to date has several limitations both general and specific to the disorder under investigation. As with all non-experimental work, it is not possible to rule out confounding or alternative explanations of associations observed between hypothesized risk factors and health outcomes of interest. With regard to alternative explanations, for example, it is noteworthy that several risk factors (e.g., socioeconomic status, neighborhood crime rates) for adverse reproductive outcomes (e.g., obstetric complications) are also independent risk factors for antisocial behavior. As a consequence, findings of an association between perinatal complications and violent criminal offending may be entirely artifactual.

Many studies measure perinatal risk with a single numerical index that combines maternal, pregnancy, obstetric, and neonatal complications. Some of these conditions pertain to the mother's health and are often present before and throughout the pregnancy (e.g., maternal chronic illness). Other adversities arise only late in gestation, at the time of labor or delivery (e.g., breach presentation). Yet others pertain to the neonate (e.g., prolonged respiratory distress). Collapsing these diverse complications into a single index creates difficulties for identifying critical periods and distinct factors in embryonic life crucial to the development of behavioral disturbance. It also obscures clues to neuropathological mechanisms and to the appropriate timing of possible intervention strategies.

We hypothesized a priori that exposure to maternal nutritional deficiency during gestation increases offspring's risk for ASPD. Early gestation as contrasted with later gestation was seen as a potentially critical period of risk since prenatal insults and toxic exposures in the 1st and 2nd trimesters had been implicated in raised rates of central nervous system anomalies and neurodevelopmental disorders (Stein et al., 1975; Kline, Stein, and Susser, 1989). In addition, minor physical anomalies originating early in gestation are reported in excess in persons with conduct disorder and aggression in childhood and violent offending in adulthood (Mednick and Kandel, 1988; Brennan, Mednick, and Kandel, 1993; Baker and Mednick, 1984; Paulus and Martin, 1986; Halverson and Victor , 1976; Waldrop et al., 1978).Nonetheless, since temporally precise understanding of embryonic development and antisocial behavior was sparse, we elected not to advance any more specific hypotheses regarding risk periods a priori (Neugebauer et al., 1999).

METHODS FOR STUDYING ANTISOCIAL PERSONALITYDISORDER

EXPOSURE

Geographic Regions and Cities

Food was rationed weekly in Holland during World War II. For rationing purposes, the government divided the country into 3 regions. The first, Western Holland, was the region where the blockade exerted its greatest force. Consequently, it is hereafter referred to as the "Famine Region". The remaining area was split into North and South, which for parsimony, we combine analytically into a single "Non-famine Region". We studied men born only in the cities throughout the Netherlands with populations exceeding 40 000 (in the Famine Region, Amsterdam, Haarlem, Leiden, Rotterdam, Utrecht and Hague) since the blockade was felt most strongly in larger urban areas (Stein et al., 1975).

Nutritional Intake .Estimates of maternal nutritional intake are based on the caloric content of the food rations and calculated for each trimester of pregnancy. Moderate nutritional deficiency is defined as mean daily rations of 1000-1500 k calories (kcal/d); severe nutritional deficiency, mean daily rations of less than 1000 kcal for the duration of a given trimester. The biological validity of the 1000 kcal/d cut point is supported by a previous finding that risk for perinatal mortality increased only at or below this level. In the Famine Region, the rations declined to less than 1000 k cal/d from February 1945 through early May 1945. Special supplements to pregnant women, available previously, were discontinued; those for infants through the first postnatal year were maintained. In the Non-Famine Region, daily rations declined to less than 1500 kcal/d but not less than 1000 kcal/d. Natural ingenuity and social privileged moderated the impact of war to some degree. Rations were enhanced by nutritional intake from other sources such as foraging for food in rural areas. The upper classes generally had more access to non-ration food than did the low classes. Nevertheless, data on fertility and other outcomes indicate a high correlation between actual food intake and official rations.

Specification of Exposures by Trimester

Men born between January 1, 1944 and December 31, 1946 inclusive are divided into 36 monthly birth cohorts. For each cohort in each region (Famine, Non-Famine) mean daily caloric content of the official ration during the 1st, 2nd and 3rd trimesters of their intrauterine life, were calculated. Moderate food deprivation occurred in both regions during 1944-1945; severe nutritional deficiency, only in the Famine Region.

Famine Region

Using the above approach, males born from February 1945 through December 1945 in the famine region (corresponding to conceptions from May 1944 through March 1945) were classified as prenatally exposed to severe nutritional deficiency. Among these individuals, men born in February, March, and April were exposed to severe nutritional deficiency in the 3rd trimester only; in May, June, and July, in the 2nd trimester only; born in August and September, in the 1st and 2nd trimesters only; born in October through December, in the 1st trimester only. Men born from September 1944 through January 1945 and in January 1946 (corresponding to conceptions from December 1943 through April 1944 and conceptions in April 1945) were classified as moderately exposed during one or more trimesters and otherwise adequately nourished. The remaining men--those born before the calendar period of moderate or severe nutritional deficiency and those conceived after these periods--were combined to form a single unexposed comparison group. The mean daily maternal food ration per trimester for these months always exceeded 1500 kcal.

Non-Famine Region

In the Non-Famine Region, men born in the north from September 1944 to November 1945 and in the south from 1944 to August 1945 were classified as prenatally exposed to moderate nutritional deficiency. The remaining monthly birth cohorts, during which maternal mean daily intake per trimester always exceeded 1500 kcal, constitute the unexposed comparison group.

MEASURE OF OUTCOME

In the 1960s, when the surviving male children born during the period 1944-1946 reached their 18th birthday, they were called up for military service and received physical, psychiatric and IQ examinations at induction centers. The examinee's date and place of birth indexed whether, to what degree and in which trimesters he was exposed to prenatal malnutrition. Linkage of any psychiatric diagnostic information with these data on date and place of birth permits a test of the association of prenatal exposure to maternal nutritional deficiency with development of ASPD by age 18 years. The diagnoses of institutionalized individuals (e.g., persons with severe mental retardation) were made based on requested medical records. Each individual could receive up to 2 diagnoses. Clergy, police, long-term prisoners, emigrants, and men with 3 older brothers who had been in the service, comprising altogether roughly 3% of potentially eligible individuals, were exempt from examination (Stein et al., 1975).

Diagnostic Criteria

Examining physicians performed psychiatric evaluations using the Dutch version of the International Classification of Diseases, Sixth Edition (ICD6) (World Health Organization, 1948; Manual of International Classification of Diseases, Injuries, and Causes of Death, Adapted 1948). While formal diagnostic criteria are not delineated in the early ICDs, descriptions of "ASPD" in Dutch psychiatric texts (Carp, 1947; Zeldenrust, 1966) from the late 1940s to the 1960s make clear that it approximates current criteria enumerated in the Diagnostic and Statistical Manual of Mental Disorders, Fourth Edition (American Psychiatric Association, 1994) ASPD was characterized by aggression, failure to conform to social norms with respect to lawful behavior (e.g., thievery and other frank criminal acts), and disregard for the truth (e.g., swindling, conning, etc.). In addition, behavioral instability and unreliability, outbursts of anger, and other interpersonal problems marked the person's childhood. In the current study persons with a primary or secondary diagnosis of ASPD constitute cases.

OTHER VARIABLES IN THE MILITARY INDUCTION EXAMINATION DATA BASE

In addition to birth date and place, the records also contain information on social class (indexed by father's occupation), IQ (i.e., Ravens Progressive Matrices), sibship size, birth order, height, and weight.

DATA ANALYSIS

The association of nutritional deficiency with ASPD was estimated using odds ratios (ORs), 95% confidence intervals (CIs), and, in multivariate analyses, maximum likelihood logistic regression (Hosmer and Lemeshow, 1989). The first analyses are conducted in the Famine Region. The odds of having ASPD among men exposed prenatally to severe nutritional deficiency and moderate nutritional deficiency are compared with the reference odds of having ASPD among men unexposed either to severe or moderate malnutrition. The second analysis is conducted in the Non-Famine Region. The odds of having ASPD among men exposed to moderate nutritional deficiency is compared with the odds among unexposed men. In the third analysis, the odds of having ASPD following severe prenatal nutritional deficiency in the Famine Region is refined further by specifying trimester(s) of exposure. Under the conditions prevailing in the current study, rarity of disease outcome, the odds ratios generated by these analyses approximates a risk ratio.

Based on a review of the published literature we identified the following potential confounding variables and other correlates of conduct disorder and ASPD: birth order, height, weight, and body mass index (BMI, calculated as weight in kilograms divided by the square of height in meters), IQ, sibship size and social class (Pine et al., 1986; Raine, 1994). Using a change of greater than 10% in the odds ratio of interest as the criterion for retaining a variable in the logistic model, only social class was a requisite covariate in the multivariable model. Both observed odds ratios and odds ratios adjusted for social class are presented in the tables while only adjusted odds ratios are discussed in the text.

In the Famine Region, an increased odds of having ASPD in severely exposed cohorts compared with unexposed cohorts might reflect a coincidental countrywide excess for the calendar period corresponding to famine exposure. We tested this question with a fourth analysis based on the entire sample of Dutch men entering terms for the main effect of region, social class, and famine exposure months, and an interaction term for region by exposure months. Specific probability values at $p<.10$ or less are reported in the text. However, in all analyses, statistical significance was set at $p<.05$.

Sample

Military examinations were conducted for 100,543 Dutch men born in Holland's larger cities (defined previously) from January 1944 to December 1946 who were residing in Holland at age 18 years. Analyses presented below pertain to this group only. (Table 1) Among the 68,932 men born in the Famine Region, 14,310 were exposed prenatally to severe nutritional deficiency during 1 or more trimesters of intrauterine life; 9615 to moderate nutritional deficiency only; 31, 45,007 were unexposed. Among the 31611 individuals born in the Non-Famine region, 10 517 were exposed prenatally to moderate nutritional deficiency; 21,094 were unexposed.

Table 1. Distribution of Men Born in Major Dutch Cities* 1944 -1946 Residing in the Netherlands at Age 18 Years by Geographic Region, Calendar Year and Prenatal Exposure to Maternal Nutritional Deficiency

Exposed (Born 1944-1946)							
Severe Exposure (<1000 kcal/d)± Trimester of Exposure:							
Geo-graphic Region	Unexposed (>1500 kcal/d, Born 1944) ++	Moderate Exposure (1000-1500kcal/d) §	1st Only	1st/ 2nd Only	2nd Only	3rd Only	Unexposed (>1500 kcal/d Born 1945 1946)^
Western Holland	13929	9615	2443	2223	4586	5058	31078
Northern / Southern Holland¶	6335	10517	…	…	…	…	14759

*Major Dutch cities comprise cities with populations exceeding 40,000 people

± Groups comprise in western Holland, men born from October through December 1945 with first-trimester exposure only, men born in August through September 1945 with first and second-trimester exposure, men born from May through July 1945 with second-trimester exposure only, and men born February through April 1945 with third-trimester exposure only

++ Groups comprise men born between January and August 1944 in western, southern and northern Holland

§ Groups comprise, in western Holland, men born from September 1944 through January 1945 and in January 1946, in northern Holland, men born from September 1944 through November 1945, and in southern Holland, men born from September 1944 through August 1945. Men born in January 1946 were exposed to moderate prenatal nutritional deficiency in the first trimester of pregnancy but were well nourished thereafter.

^Groups comprise, in western Holland, men born from February through December 1946, in northern Holland, men born from December 1945 through December 1946, in southern Holland, men born from September 1945 through December 1946.

In northern Holland, 2761, 4889, and 6154 were unexposed in 1944, moderately exposed in 1944-1945, and unexposed in 1945-1946, respectively. The corresponding figures in southern Holland were 3574, 5628, and 8605. Ellipses indicate persons that residing in northern and southern Holland were not exposed to severe nutritional deficiency.

RESULTS

In the Famine Region, the odds of ASPD were elevated among men with severe but not with moderate prenatal nutritional deficiency. The adjusted odds ratios were 2.0 (95% CI 1.2-3.3) and 0.7 (0.3-1.6), respectively (Table 2) These individuals in the Famine Region were sub-grouped further by trimester of exposure to severe nutritional deficiency (Table 3) to examine whether the increased odds of ASPD applied equally throughout gestation, varied by trimester or was possibly confined to only one or two trimesters. Odds ratios for 1st and/or 2nd-trimester exposures ranged from 2.1 to 3.0 and did not differ significantly from each other. The odds of ASPD were not increased as a consequence of exposure to third-trimester nutritional deficiency. (The difference in odds between 1st and/or 2nd-trimester exposure and third-trimester exposure was statistically significant at P<.10.)

Table 2. Association Between Antisocial Personality Disorder (ASPD) in Dutch Men atAge 18 Years and Moderate or Severe Prenatal Nutritional Deficiency: WesternHolland (Famine Region), 1944-1946

Level of Nutritional Deficiency*	Population N	Cases of ASPD N	Prevalence of ASPD per 10,000	OR (95% CL), Observed/Adjusted±
Severe (<1000 kcal/d)	14310	26	18.2	1.6 (1.02-2.6)/2.0 (1.2-3.3)
Moderate (1000-1500 kcal/d)	9615	10	10.4	0.9 (0.6-1.9)/0.7 (0.3-1.6)
Unexposed (>1500 kJcal/d)	45007	50	11.1	Reference

*Value pertains to average daily rations during 1 or more trimesters of pregnancy. For

calendar birth dates corresponding to exposure categories, see "Methods" section of text.

± OR indicates odds ratio; CI, confidence interval, ORs to the right of the virgules are adjusted for social class (manual laborers including farmers and nonmanual laborers). The comparison between the odds of antisocial personality disorder associated with moderate vs severe exposure is statistically significant; the comparison between the moderately exposed and unexposed is not

Table 3. Association Between Antisocial Personality Disorder and Severe Prenatal Nutritional Deficiency in Dutch Men at Age 18 Years Over and by Trimester of Exposure: Western Holland (Famine Region), 1944-1946

Trimester of Exposure*	Population N	Cases of ASPD N	Prevalence of ASPD per 10,000	OR (95% CI), Observed/Adjusted ±
1, 2, or 3	14310	26	18.2	1.6 (1.02-2.6)/2.0 (1.2-3.3)
1 and/or 2	9252	20	21.6	2.0 (1.2-3.5)/2.5 (1.5-4.2)
1 only	2443	6	24.6	2.2 (0.95-5.0)/2.9 (1.2-6.7)
1 and 2 only	2223	6	27.0	2.4 (1.04-5.7)/3.0 (1.3-7.0)
2 only	4586	9	19.6	1.8 (0.9-3.6)/2.1(1.03-4.4)
3 only	5058	5	9.9	0.9 (0.4-2.2)/1.1 (0.4-2.7)
Unexposed	45007	50	11.1	Reference

*Values pertain to average daily rations during 1 or more trimesters of pregnancy. For calendar birth dates corresponding to exposure categories, see "Methods" section of text.

±OR indicates odds ration; CI, confidence interval. ORs to the right of the virgules are adjusted for social class (manual laborers (including farmers) and nonmanual laborers).

In the Non-Famine Region, the odds of ASPD was not associated with moderate nutritional deficiency (adjusted OR, 1.0; 95% CI, 0.6-1.7). In a nation wide analysis the elevated odds of having ASPD was restricted to men born in the Famine Region exposed to severe nutritional deficiency. Individuals conceived in the Non-Famine Region during the same calendar period of the blockade at its severest point, but unexposed to severe maternal nutritional deficiency, did not exhibit increased rates of ASPD. Thus, the excess ASPD rate was confined to the Famine Region and the calendar period of severe nutritional deficiency.

Schizophrenia

BACKGROUND

Our schizophrenia investigation (Susser, Neugebauer and Hoek, 1996) predated and served as the template for the work on ASPD. The neurodevelopmental hypothesis of the etiology of schizophrenia, like that for ASPD, posits that a disruption of early brain development produced in the prenatal or perinatal period exercises a causal role in a substantial proportion of schizophrenia cases. This hypothesis is supported by converging evidence from a variety of fields, including longitudinal studies of high risk offspring and research on neuro-imagining and neuropathology (Marenco and Weinberger, 2000; Murray, Jones, Susser, Van Os and Cannon, 2003).

If the interval from conception to birth comprises a period of biological vulnerability to factors that influence risk for schizophrenia, what particular factors warrant attention? A host of plausible risk factors have been advanced, in addition to the nutritional hypothesis considered here, including season of birth, i.e., an excess of winter/spring births; Rhesis incompatibility; obstetric complications as well as certain neonatal infections (Cannon, Kendell, Susser, Jones, 2003).

Two other factors warrant brief separate mention: prenatal infection and maternal stress. Suspected prenatal infectious, notably viral, etiologies have a long pedigree. Most studies have demonstrated that individuals in utero during influenza epidemics evidence increased rates of schizophrenia, with 2nd trimester exposure contributing most to these results. Rubella, a known cause of neurodevelopmental anomalies and a risk factor for autism, has been implicated in our own recent work in risk for non-affective psychosis, including schizophrenia (Susser, Brown and Matte, 1999; Brown et al., 2004).

Three studies of the potential role of prenatal maternal stress in the etiology of schizophrenia in offspring are especially noteworthy in the current context. One investigation reported increased risk for schizophrenia among the posthumous children of men who died in the Russo-Finnish war in 1939 (Huttenen and Niskanen, 1978); a second, increased risk for schizophrenia among individuals in utero at the time of the May 1940 German invasion of the Netherlands (Van Os and Selden, 1998); a third, increased risk for schizophrenia associated with prenatal exposure to a severe tornado (Kinney, Hyman, Geetham and Tramer, 1999) Extensive animal literature affords evidence that prenatal maternal stress alters fetal brain development and subsequent offspring behavior (Suomi, 1997), an effect thought to be mediated by the impact of glucocorticoid on the fetal hypothalamo-pituitary-adrenal axis (Cannon, Kendell, Susser, Jones, 2003) However, stress-related depressed appetite and consequent reduction in food intake associated with bereavement (in the case of the Finnish study) or with distress generally might also contribute to these findings.

METHODS FOR STUDYING SCHIZOPHRENIA AND FAMINE

The methods of determining kcal/d, applying these values to trimesters, and the division into Famine and Non-Famine Regions are the same as in the study of ASPD, both patterned on Stein et al. (1975).

EXPOSURE

Geographic Regions and Cities

Preliminary work on famine and schizophrenia (Susser and Lin, 1992) investigated the possible impact of prenatal exposure to varying degrees of maternal nutritional deficiency in the Famine and Non-Famine Regions. Given space limitations here we focus exclusively on the subsequent, definitive elaboration of findings for the Famine Region only.

Refinement of Exposure Criteria: Restriction by Severity and Trimester

The identification of the 1st and 2nd trimesters of gestation as critical periods for the later development of ASPD, while striking, was nonetheless largely post hoc. By contrast, previous work examining neurodevelopmental hypotheses for schizophrenia enabled us to proceed with a more precise a prior hypothesis regarding both the timing and the degree of the prenatal nutritional insult. Consequently, we were able to formulate a strict exposure algorithm.

Three criteria were used to define exposed birth cohorts: (1) low maternal food rations during the 1st trimester of intrauterine life, (2) conception at the height of the famine, and (3) increased frequency of congenital neural defects among individuals comprising the cohort. Regarding the first criterion, average food rations during the 1st trimester were below 1000 kcal/d for individuals born between August and December 1945. These cohorts were defined as exposed to low rations. All other birth cohorts were defined as unexposed. For the second criterion, we relied on the documented health outcomes of the famine period, indicating that the height of the famine was toward the end of the Hunger Winter (February through April 1945). The population was nutritionally depleted, and the effects on morbidity and mortality most severe (Stein et al., 1975; Burger, Drummond, and Sandstead, 1947). Among the cohorts of August through December 1945, only the later born (October 15 through December 31, 1945) were conceived during the height of the famine and, therefore, also met our second criterion for exposure. We shall refer to these later born as the EX2 cohort. The earlier born (August 1 through October 14, 1945) were conceived in the early months of the Hunger Winter and did not meet our second criterion for exposure. Owing to the timing of their conception, the EX2 cohort was marked by fertility below 50% of previous levels; the EX1 cohort suffered a smaller decline in fertility.

With regard to the third exposure criterion, we computed the risk in the EX2, EX1 and unexposed cohorts for congenital neural defects with established or strongly suspected links with early prenatal nutritional deficiency. (For details on databases and computational methods employed in these analyses see Susser et al., 1975.) The EX2 cohort had a detectable excess of congenital neural defects, while the EX1 cohort did not exhibit any such excess. Examination of secular trends for the entire period 1944-46 also provided compelling evidence of a pronounced peak in risk for congenital neural defects in the EX2 cohort. Thus, the exposed birth cohorts comprised two distinct groups: the EX2 cohort which met all three exposure criteria's the EX1 cohort met only one of the three criteria.

OUTCOME

Since the median age of onset for schizophrenia is in the 20's, the military induction examination data were not useful for investigation of this outcome. Consequently, we utilized the Dutch National psychiatric registry to ascertain cases of schizophrenia for the proposed analyses. At the time of our study, registry data were available for 1970 through 1992, comprising persons 24 to 48 years of age for the birth cohorts of 1944 through 1946. Data on cases were derived from psychiatric and university hospitals, which account for more than 90% of psychiatric admissions in the Netherlands. Data on each case included ICD-8-ICD-9 (World Health Organization, 1938) diagnosis, place of birth, and week of birth.

Two definitions of schizophrenia were employed: narrow and broad. "Narrowly defined" included only those cases in which the ICD-8ICD-9 diagnosis was that of paranoid, hebephrenic, residual, or catatonic schizophrenia,' in accordance with the modern criteria for the disorder (American Psychiatric Association, 1994). While severely limiting the number of cases available for analysis, this definition reduced the risk of misclassifying affective psychoses as schizophrenia. "Broadly defined" comprised all cases with an ICD-9 diagnosis of schizophrenia, irrespective of the subtype. Individuals were classified based on their most recent discharge diagnosis.

OTHER VARIABLES IN THE DUTCH PSYCHIATRIC REGISTRY DATA BASE

For each case reported by the registry, the only data provided were the birth date, birth place, gender, number and date of each psychiatric admission and diagnosis at each admission.

DATA ANALYSIS

The risks for schizophrenia in the EX2 cohort, the EX I cohort, and the unexposed cohort were computed by dividing the number of schizophrenia cases by the number of births minus deaths up to age 18 years in each cohort. Each quotient was expressed as a cumulative incidence per 1000 persons. Relative risks (RR) were calculated together with 95% CLs (Fleiss, 1981). The chi-square statistic was used to test the null hypothesis of no association between exposure and disease. Seasonal and other fluctuations in the rate of schizophrenia were examined by dividing the birth cohorts of 1944-46 into smaller cohorts, each of 2 months duration. However, to maintain the integrity of the EX 1 and EX2 cohorts, the period of May through December 1945 was divided into just three periods: May through July, August 1 through October 14 (EX1), and October 15 through December 31 (EX2). (For further details regarding both the rationale and mechanics of these computations see Susser, Neugebauer and Hoek, 1996)

Sample

The entire study cohort comprised 146,347 individuals with 93.4% classified as unexposed to severe prenatal malnutrition in their 1st trimester. Among the remaining individuals, 2.9% were in the EX1 cohort (n=5466) and 3.7% in the EX2 (n=4190) cohort.

RESULTS

With regard to narrowly defined schizophrenia, risk was significantly higher in the EX2 cohort than in the unexposed cohort (Table 4) (RR=2.0; 95% CI = 1.2 to 3.4; P<.01). The RR did not vary by gender; among men, the RR=1.9 (95% Cl = 1.0 to 3.7; P=.05), and among women, the RR = 2.2 (95% Cl = 1.0 to 4.7; P=.04). The risk for schizophrenia was not increased in the EX1 cohort. The Figure shows the risk for schizophrenia in 17 successive two month birth cohorts of 1944 through 1946. The risk for schizophrenia peaked in the EX2 cohort and was otherwise stable.

We reanalyzed the finding for the EX2 cohort under a broad definition of schizophrenia and using other procedures for selecting the diagnosis. The association between early prenatal exposure to famine and schizophrenia was consistent under six approaches.

Table 4. Schizophrenia* in Birth Cohorts Exposed± and Unexposed± to Early Prenatal Nutritional Deficiency During the Dutch Hunger Winter of 1944 Through 1945: Cumulative Incidence Data

Level of Nutritional Deficiency Total	Population N	Cumulative Incidencper 1000 persons++(	e N cases) Relative risk at age 24-48 y (95% CI) P
EX 2	4190	3.8 (16)	2.0 (1.2 – 3.4) <.01
EX 1	5466	2.0 (11)	1.1 (0.6 – 2.0) .82
Unexposed	136,691	1.9 (257)	
Men			
EX 2	2184	4.1 (9)	1.9 (1.0-3.7) .05
EX 1	2800	2.5 (7)	1.2 (0.5-2.5) .70
Unexposed	69,943	2.2 (151)	

Table 4. (Continued)

Women			
EX 2	2006	3.5 (7)	2.2 (1.0-4.7) .04
EX 1	2666	1.5 (4)	0.9 (0.4-2.6) .91
Unexposed	68,748	1.6 (106)	

*Schizophrenia narrowly defined, ie, ICD-9 (International Classification of Diseases, Ninth Revision) 295.1,2,3,6.

± EX2 indicates exposed birth cohort of October 15 through December 31, 1945; EX1, exposed birth cohort of August 1 through October 14, 1945; and unexposed, all other births of 1944 through 1946 in famine cities.

++ Denominators are live births minus deaths up to age 18 years

1944-1946

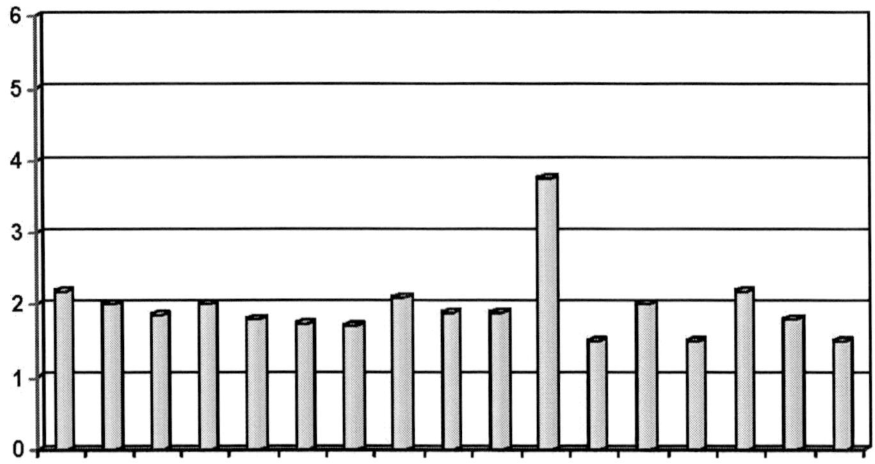

Jan-FebMar-AprMay-JunJul-Aug Sep-OctNov-DecJan-Feb

Mar-Apr

May-Jul EX1EX2

Jan-FebMar-AprMay-JunJul-Aug Sep-OctNov-Dec

Figure 1. Schizophrenia in adulthood (hospitalized cases of 24 to 48 years of age) in Dutch birth cohorts of 1944 through 1946. EX1 and EX2 represent cohorts born August 1 - October 14, 1945, and October 15 - December 31, 1945, respectively; bar, 95% confidence limits

SUMMARY OF FINDINGS FOR ANTISOCIAL PERSONALITY DISORDER AND SCHIZOPHRENIA

These studies offer evidence of a relationship between early prenatal nutritional deficiency and the risk for ASPD and for schizophrenia in offspring. The ASPD findings suggest that exposure to severe nutritional deficiency in the 1st and/or 2nd trimesters of intrauterine life is associated with a 2-3 fold increased risk for development of ASPD among males. Exposure at other times and to only moderate nutritional deficiency does not confer risk. No information was available on this question for females. The schizophrenia findings suggest that exposure early in gestation at the height of the Dutch Hunger Winter (EX2) doubled risk for schizophrenia both in males and females. This increased risk was evident under all definitions of schizophrenia, but most marked under a narrow definition consistent with modern criteria. Taken together, the notable specificity in these outcomes and in the exposure enhances the credibility of these findings for both disorders.

STRENGTH OF THE STUDY DESIGN

The origin of the nutritional exposure under study in a large-scale, geographically and temporally delimited historical conflict, driven by forces extrinsic to those that pattern disease in Dutch society, confers several methodological and inferential strengths on these findings.

First, the Dutch Hunger Winter permits an examination of the effect of a relatively specific antenatal insult--nutritional deprivation. Second, the timing of the exposure in prenatal development can be identified with unique precision. Third, the community-wide nature of the exposure and its imposition by military force created a quasi-experimental condition likely to reduce the effect of potentially confounding factors.

Pursuing the example of potential confounding offered at the outset of this chapter, in peacetime low socioeconomic status is a risk factor for adverse reproductive outcomes such as birth complications which have been implicated in violent criminal offending in adulthood. Low socioeconomic status is also a risk factor for antisocial behavior. An observed association between birth complications and antisocial behavioral therefore may be an artifact of confounding. By contrast, the specific risk factor under study here—severe nutritional deficiency—was introduced by foreign blockade whose distribution, timing and to a large degree intensity was governed by forces acting entirely independent of the class structure of Dutch society. Fourth, the absence of severe nutritional deficiency in the Non-Famine Region allows a test of whether the increased odds of developing ASPD or schizophrenia reflected some countrywide rise in 1944-45 unrelated to the nutritional crisis. Finally, the restriction of the sample to 18-year old men in the ASPD analysis eliminated an extraneous source of variance, i.e., age, in the dependent measure, thereby affording a more precise estimate of effect.

REPLICATION OF THE DUTCH FAMINE SCHIZOPHRENIA FINDINGS:STUDY OF THE CHINESE FAMINE 1959-61

A recent study of schizophrenia among persons exposed in utero to the Chinese Famine that occurred in 1959-61 offers a substantial and important replication of the Dutch results

(St. Clair, Zu, Wang , Yu, Fang, Zhang, Zheng, Gu, Feng, Sham , He , 2005). Among persons born in a famine-affected region in China 1960, the adjusted relative risk for schizophrenia (based on psychiatric hospital inpatient and outpatient data) was 2.30 (95% CI 1.99-2.65). These results, based on altogether different historical and cultural circumstances, afford strong independent confirmation of the neurodevelopmental and specifically prenatal nutritional hypothesis for schizophrenia. Further details of the Chinese work, as it helps to address certain limitations in the original Dutch findings, are discussed below.

LIMITATIONS

Ecological Nature of the Measurement of Exposure

Despite the strengths of the Dutch study several limitations--both intrinsic to our study design and to observational studies generally—prompt some caution in accepting these results. A primary limitation is the ecological measurement of nutritional status. The nutritional status of individual pregnant women was not directly measured but was based on official government food rations. Redistribution of food rations within households, supplementation from the black market, or foraging in the countryside could introduce misclassification into our estimates. Considerable evidence from different sources indicates that whatever the degree of misclassification, it enjoyed sufficient true variance to achieve discernable effects. Other studies of these birth cohorts document associations between famine exposure, measured ecologically, and immediate reproductive and intergenerational health outcomes (Ravelli et al., 1976; Ravelli et al., 1998; Lumey, Stein and Ravelli, 1995; Susser and Lin, 1992; Hoek et al., 1996; Brown et al, 1995; Brown and Susser, 1997). Macro level historical data confirm the near ubiquity of the famine for urban populations. Furthermore, while the famine's force varied somewhat by social class, (Susser, Neugebauer and Hoek, 1998) reflecting the fact that even calamities can become socialized, this differential is adjusted for in our analyses of ASPD and did not require adjustment in the case of schizophrenia.

Doubts attending the ecological measurement of exposure are further defused by the Chinese findings, despite the fact that it also utilized an ecological measure of nutritional intake. By replicating the Dutch findings under vastly different historical conditions, the Chinese results reduce the likelihood that some third factor, coinciding with but distinct from the famine, accounts for the association of nutritional deprivation with schizophrenia risk. Furthermore, the far greater severity, extent and duration of the Chinese famine, involving an 80% decline in birth rate, makes it extremely unlikely that more privileged social groups in the population escaped the famine's force and operated as a confounder in the analysis. Hence, the consistency of the Chinese and Dutch results reinforce our premise that ecologically measured and individual level nutritional intake are highly correlated under famine conditions, a conclusion that also serves to strengthen the ASPD findings.

Dates of conception were also not directly measured, producing error in the assignment of individuals to exposure category. However, neither random misspecification of exposure status nor of timing of exposure would threaten the validity of our positive findings. Rather, such measurement errors would produce underestimates, not overestimates, of risk (Rothman and Greenland, 1998).

Other limitations of the schizophrenia study included the use of registry diagnoses, the absence of patients younger than 24 years of age, and, for both investigations, the loss to emigration of a small number of cohort members. Because each of these factors would likely affect the exposed and unexposed cohorts in the same way, they would not account for the reported associations. Rather, they would tend to diminish the observed association owing to nondifferential misclassification.

OTHER NEURODEVELOPMENTAL TOXINS AND VIRAL ETIOLOGIES

Famine could lead to eating of food substitutes, e.g., tulip bulbs, constitute a severe stressor affecting prenatal maternal hormones, (Huttenen and Niskanen, 1978) and was followed by rapid nutritional repletion with the Allied victory. In theory these exposures could exert toxic effects on the developing brain.

Finally, a thorough search was undertaken to locate evidence of non-nutritional exposures that coincided with the height of the famine in the Netherlands and that could account for our findings. None were identified. It is true that a nationwide rise in infant infections, including tuberculosis, typhoid and dysentery, occurred in the months afterward (Stein et al., 1975). Arguably, one or more of these conditions could have played an etiologic role in one or both of the conditions studies. However, none of these factors followed a temporal or geographic pattern that could account for effects that were restricted to the Famine region and to the first two trimesters of pregnancy. Hence, they are unsatisfactory as competing explanatory factors. The Chinese results, arising of course in the absence of tulip bulb consumption and characterized by a very gradual recovery from starvation, further diminishes the reasonableness of any of these competing explanations.

DIAGNOSTIC VALIDITY AND CASE ASCERTAINMENT

Antisocial Personality Disorder

Clinical descriptions of ASPD in the 1960s readily concur with current criteria and the descriptive epidemiology of this entity in the military data, e.g., inverse relationship with social class, affords evidence of constructive validity. However, given the relatively low frequency of this diagnosis among recruits, it is reasonable to conclude both that ASPD was under diagnosed and the individuals so diagnosed comprised the more severe cases.

Case Ascertainment Unbiased by the Criminal Justice System

In many studies of ASPD and of criminal offending more generally, cases comprise individuals arrested or arrested and successfully prosecuted for criminal behavior. Such individuals, while typical of one segment of the prison population, are unlikely to be representative of antisocial individuals in general. Additionally, some cases will in fact be innocent of the commission of a crime. Therefore, risk factors identified in such studies may represent risk for detection, arrest and conviction rather than for the commission of antisocial acts per se. Hence, strength of the current study is that it achieves case ascertainment largely independently of the individual's relationship to the legal system.

The one exception to this statement pertains to long-term prisoners --many probably meeting criteria for ASPD (Kaplan and Sadock,1991) – who were exempt from military induction. However, few 18-year-old Dutch men are likely to fall into this category. Moreover, any unascertained cases of ASPD would only threaten the validity of our positive findings if length of incarceration were directly associated with 1st- and/or 2nd-trimester exposure. Unbiased case under ascertainment per se will not inflate the OR (Rothman and Greenland, 1998)

Schizophrenia

The schizophrenia findings rely on the use of hospitalized cases of the disorder. Consequently, the question arises as to whether the apparent increased risk for schizophrenia reflects simply an increased likelihood of ascertainment and hospitalization of cases exposed to famine early in gestation. Apart from the inherent implausibility of such a specific bias in hospitalization patterns, two independent findings further reduce the reasonableness of this alternative explanation. First, Chinese famine results derived from a study of outpatient and inpatient cases, thereby requiring that the bias in hospitalization patterns also extended to outpatient care. Second, conception at the height of the Dutch famine has also been implicated in increased risk for schizophrenia spectrum personality disorder, a finding based on the same military data as were employed in the ASPD analyses(Hoek, Susser, Buck, Lumey, Lin, and Gorman,1996). Diagnoses in the military records are entirely independent of treatment status and hence, free of any possible bias pertaining to entry into treatment. These results for schizoid personality disorder help to counter the concerns raised here regarding reliance on treated cases of schizophrenia.

SELECTION BIAS

Selective Conception

Did couples at elevated risk of having antisocial offspring enjoy superior fertility under famine conditions? If so, the apparent association between ASPD and famine could be artifactual. For example, sociopathic parents might circumvent equitable official food rationing, thereby securing a reproductive advantage over more rule bound couples. However, fertility was most affected by nutritional deficiency at time of conception and mortality in the first year of life was most affected by nutritional deficiency in the third trimester. Thus, such differential fertility, even if present, cannot explain the increased risk of ASPD associated with 2nd trimester famine exposure. More simply, the excess rate of offspring with ASPD and reproductive advantage among such couples would have to be extraordinarily high to have an appreciable impact on the adjusted ORs.

Selective conception is also unlikely to account for the schizophrenia findings. Hypothetically, individuals carrying susceptibility alleles for schizophrenia might be more inclined to maintain efforts at conception during the famine. Poor nutrition was probably the most critical factor influencing conception. Therefore, we would expect such women to have reduced conception rates because they were less effective in competing for black market and other extra food rations.

Selective Survival

Live births in the exposed cohorts comprise conceptions that survived arduous intrauterine circumstances. It has been argued that schizophrenia's persistence in the population, despite reduced fertility and survival of affected individuals, may be explained by the relevant genes conferring a selective survival advantage in some contexts, for example, in the context of fetal wastage owing to severe malnutrition. An analogous causal model could be advanced for ASPD, which is also characterized by increased adult mortality rates for affected individuals. However, at present, no evidence is available to directly support this causal model.

The Chinese famine study investigated this question of selective reproduction directly by examining the frequency of mental disorder among the family members of cases. The proportion of cases having relatives with psychiatric illness did not differ among those born before, during or after the famine years, a result that diminishes the plausibility of the selective procreation hypothesis (St. Clair, Zu, Wang , Yu, Fang, Zhang, Zheng, Gu, Feng, Sham , He , 2005). However, the absence of comparisons specific to schizophrenia and the unreliability of family history data generally mean that appreciable differences in genetic susceptibility to schizophrenia might still be present but obscured by measurement error (Neugebauer, 2005).

MEDIATING MECHANISMS

As previously noted, obstetric complications have been associated both with an increased risk for ASPD and for schizophrenia. Therefore, prenatal nutritional deficiency may have exerted its pathogenic effects indirectly though such perinatal complications. Individual level data to test this proposed mediating mechanism are unfortunately not available. However, perinatal complications are reflected in perinatal mortality rates and these rates were elevated among famine births. However, some of the unexposed birth cohorts of 1944-1946 were also afflicted by high perinatal mortality, for other reasons, yet these cohorts did not experience elevated rates of ASPD or schizophrenia.

Pregnancy complications may compromise maternal-child interactions, for example, by raising maternal or offspring risk for physical illness, thereby increasing offspring's risk for behavioral problems (Cohler et al., 1975; Robinson and Robinson, 1965; Field et al., 1986; Grigoroiu-Servanescu, 1984; McGee et al., 1984). However, the similarity in rates of physical morbidity between exposed cases and exposed noncases, together with the absence of a 3rd trimester effect of severe nutritional deficiency on the outcomes studied, renders these proposed intervening mechanisms implausible. Finally, the excess of ASPD among exposed cohorts is not explained by an independent effect of nutritional deficiency on measured physical illness, depressed IQ, sibship size, or BMI.

LIMITATIONS ON GENERALIZABILITY OF FINDINGS

Assuming adequate internal validity for these findings, to what extent can these results be generalized beyond our samples? Regarding our ASPD findings for 18 year olds males, we do not know whether they apply to antisocial behavior of prepubital origin, (Lyons et al., 1995) or to women. Furthermore, estimations of the magnitude of the contribution of prenatal factors to antisocial behavior is necessarily relativistic. In certain social environments (e.g., communities characterized by high concentrations of economic disadvantage, political disenfranchisement, and limited "collective efficacy" (Sampson, Raudenbush and Earls, 1997)) postnatal risk factors may dwarf the independent role of prenatal ones.

Early prenatal nutritional deficiency could produce the observed effects either because of general malnutrition or of a specific micronutrient deficiency. Severe prenatal protein-calorie malnutrition is a rare exposure that occurs mainly in developing countries. In developed countries, it could account only for a small number of cases in special circumstances. A specific prenatal micronutrient deficiency, on the other hand, might play an important role in developed as well as in developing countries (Stein et al., 1975; Baker and Mednick, 1984; Paulus and Martin, 1986).

The findings for neural tube defects such as spina bifida and anencephaly exemplify this point. Early prenatal folate deficiency has remained an important causative factor for neural tube defects in wealthy societies. The incidence appears to depend on the specific micronutrient composition of the diet, and on the genetic background of the population, rather than on overall food intake, and it follows no simple gradient across rich and poor societies.

These findings may also have implications for societies that are victimized by ongoing civil wars. The Dutch Hunger Winter imposed conditions of severe nutritional deficiency on a population that was reasonably well nourished prior to the blockade and in its immediate aftermath. The implications of these findings for developing countries, where episodes of maternal starvation, often associated with civil war, natural disaster, forced migration, and refugee status (Neugebauer, 1997) are superimposed on conditions of endemic under nutrition, await clarification. Future efforts at replication and extension of these results to more heterogeneous samples, including samples in developing countries, are needed

While we conclude that prenatal nutritional deficiency offers the most compelling and parsimonious explanation for these findings, a prenatal nutritional contribution to risk for ASPD and schizophrenia does not preclude or outrank other explanatory factors; indeed, it may depend upon other factors to exert appreciable effects.. With regard to the ASPD findings, we note that the results for 1st and/or 2nd-trimester nutritional deficiency are compatible with separate genetic and pregnancy or postnatal environmental contributions to risk. The folate model proposed above for schizophrenia is suitable here as well. Periconceptional nutritional deficiency increases risk for neural tube defects but possibly only or primarily among genetically at-risk individuals (Elwood, Little and Elwood, 1992). On the other hand, nutritional deficiency early in pregnancy may enhance fetal susceptibility to obstetric insults. Furthermore, these findings do not preclude a substantial contribution of poverty, social disadvantage, and early family environment to the development of antisocial behaviors, especially because maternal nutritional deficiency reflects in part the prenatal operation of social and economic forces. Finally, intrauterine factors can mimic genetic patterns of disease transmission. Therefore, identification of intrauterine factors in offspring's risk for antisocial behavior may improve estimation and specification of possible genetic contributions, an issue whose place in history and current politics is naturally highly charged (Gershon, 1995).

With regard to the schizophrenia findings we note that prenatal nutritional deficiency could act in conjunction with either genetic factors or other prenatal exposures (Susser, Neugebauer and Hoek, 1996). In this regard too, neural tube defects may serve as a useful paradigm. These defects are influenced by genetic factors, as well as by prenatal nutrition, and comprise several types that may be genetically distinct. Recent findings, that in the presence of an impairment in homocysteine metabolism, which may be genetically determined, a higher than average periconceptional intake of vitamin B_{12} or of folate may compensate by overcoming the metabolic defect and, thereby, reduce the risk for neural tube defects in offspring.

Advances in our knowledge of DNA methylation now make folic acid a candidate micronutrient, not just an exemplar, in efforts to understand nutrition and schizophrenia. Levels in the diet of methyl-donor components, for example, of folic acid, affect DNA methylation. In turn DNA methylation at cystosines in cytosine guanine dinucleotides can alter gene expression and functioning without perturbing the primary DNA sequence (Neugebauer, 2005). Recent research documents a role for such DNA-methylation alternations in DNA expression early in development and also in several adult-onset disorders. In a 2005 meta-analysis, Lewis and colleagues (Lewis, Zammit, Gunnell and Smith, 2005) found a link between the MTHFR C677T genotype, known to exercise a role in folate metabolism, with risk for schizophrenia, thereby identifying a direct connection between folate metabolism and the intracellular availability of folate metabolites for methylation with the development of schizophrenia. These results, while still preliminary, support our conceptualization of schizophrenia as a genetic neurodevelopmental disorder that may entail prenatal nutritional alternation of gene expression. The distant possibility is raised, therefore, of primary prevention strategies for this most destructive of psychiatric disorders.

CONCLUSION

The strength of the reported associations, the security of the temporal order, specificity of 1st- and/or 2nd trimester effect, and the coherence with findings in collateral research support the view that early prenatal nutritionally related insults to the developing brain are implicated as risk factors for antisocial behavior and schizophrenia. Much future work is required to identify the specific mechanisms of action by which particular nutritional deficiencies operate at precise stages of embryonic development to achieve such devastating and crippling impediments to normal human development.

REFERENCES

American Psychiatric Association. (1994). Diagnostic and Statistical Manual of Mental Disorders. (4th ed.). Washington, DC: American Psychiatric Association.

Baker, R.L., Mednick, B.R. (1984). Influences on Human Development: A Longitudinal Perspective. Boston: Kluwer-Nijhoff.

Barker, D.J. (2003a). Commentary: Developmental origins of raised serum cholesterol. International Journal of Epidemiology, 32, 876-877.

Barker, D.J. (2003b). The developmental origins of adult disease. European Journal of Epidemiology, 18, 733-736.

Brennan, P., Mednick, S.A., Kandel, E. (1993). Congenital determinants of violent and property offending. In D.J. Pepler and K.H. Rubin (Eds). The Development and Treatment of Childhood Aggression (pp. 81-92). Hillsdale, NJ: Lawrence Erlbaum Associates.

Brown, A., Susser, E., Lin, S.P., Neugebauer, R. and Gorman, J.M. (1995). Increased risk for affective disorders in males after second trimester prenatal exposure to the Dutch Hunger Winter of 1944-45. British Journal of Psychiatry, 166, 601-606.

Brown, A.S., Begg, M.D., Gravenstein, S., Schaefer, C.A., Wyatt, R.J., Bresnahan, M., Babulas, V.P., Susser, E.S. (2004). Serologic evidence of prenatal influenza in the etiology of schizophrenia. Archives of General Psychiatry, 61, 774-780.

Brown, A.S. and Susser, E.S. (1997). Sex differences in prevalence of congenital neural defects after periconception famine exposure. Epidemiology, 8, 555-558.

Burger, G.C.E., Drummond, J.C.,and Sandstead, H.R.,(Eds). (1947) Malnutrition and Starvation in the Western Netherlands: September 1944-July 1945. The Hague: General Printing Office.

Cannon M, Kendell R, Susser E and Jones P. (2003). Chapter 5. Prenatal and perinatal risk factors for schizophrenia. IN The Epidemiology of Schizophrenia. Eds Murray RM, Jones PBN, Susser E and Van Os J, Cannon M. (2003) Cambridge University Press, London. Chapter 5, pp. 74-99.

Carp, E.A.D.E. (1947). Medische Psychologie en Pathopsychologie. Part 3. Amsterdam: Scheltema and Holkema.

Cohler, B.J., Gallant, D.H., Gruenbaum, H.U., Weiss, J.L. and Gamer, E. (1975). Pregnancy and birth complications among mentally ill and well mothers and their children. Social Biology, 22, 269-277.

Diagnostic and Statistical Manual of Mental Disorders, Fourth Edition.(1994). Washington, DC: American Psychiatric Press;

Elwood, J.M., Little, J. and Elwood, J.H. (1992). Epidemiology and Control of Neural Tube Defects. New York: Oxford University Press.

Field, T.M., Sandberg, D., Garcia, R., Vega-Lahr, N., Goldstein, S., and Guy, L. (1985). Pregnancy problems, postpartum depression, and early mother-infant interactions. Developmental Psychology, 21, 1152-1156.

Gershon, E.S. (1995). Antisocial behavior. Archives of General Psychiatry, 52, 900-901.

Grigoroiu-Servanescu, M. (1984). Intellectual and emotional development and school adjustment in preterm children at 6 and 7 years of age. International Journal of Behavioral Development, 7, 307-320.

Halverson, C.F. and Victor, J.B. (1976). Minor physical anomalies and problem behavior in elementary school children. Child Development, 47, 281-285.

Harding, J.E. (2001). The nutritional basis of the fetal origins of adult disease. International Journal of Epidemiology, 30, 15-23.

Hoek, H.W., Susser, E., Buck, K.A., Lumey, L.H., Lin, S.P., Gorman, J.M. (1996). Schizoid personality disorder after prenatal exposure to famine. American Journal of Psychiatry, 153, 1637-1639.

Hosmer, D.W. and Lemeshow, S. (1989). Applied Logistic Regression. New York: John Wiley and Sons Inc.

Huttenen, M. and Niskanen, P. (1978). Prenatal loss of father and psychiatric disorders. Archives of General Psychiatry, 35, 429-431. International Journal of Epidemiology (2001) 30.

Kaplan, H.I., and Sadock, B.J. (Eds.). (1991). Personality disorders. In: Synopsis of Psychiatry. (6th ed.).

Kinney DK, Hyman W, Greetham C and Tramer S. (1999). Increased relative risk for schizophrenia and prenatal exposure to a severe tornado. Schizophrenia Research 36: 45-46. Kline, J, Stein, Z. and Susser, M. (1989). Conception to Birth: Epidemiology of Prenatal Development. New York: Oxford University Press. Leon, D.A. (2001). Commentary: Getting to grips with fetal programming-aspects of a rapidly evolving agenda. International Journal of Epidemiology, 30, 96-98.

Lewis SJ, Zammit S, Gunnell D and Smith GD. (2005). A meta-analysis of the MTHFR C677T polymorphism and schizophrenia risk. Am J Med Genet B Neuropsychiatr Genet. 135, 2-4.

Lumey, L.H., Stein, A.D., Ravelli, A.C. (1995). Timing of prenatal starvation in women and birth weight in their first and second born offspring. European Journal of Obstetrics, Gynecology and Reproductive Biology, 61, 23-30.

Lyons, M.J., True, W.R., Eisen, S.A., et al. (1995). Differential heritability of adult and juvenile antisocial traits. Archives of General Psychiatry. 52: 906-915.

Manual of the International Classification of Diseases, Injuries and Causes of Death, Sixth Revision [translated and edited for the Netherlands in 6 decimals by Dr. I.J. van der Mandele]. Adapted 1948.

Marenco S, Weinberger DR. (2000). The neurodevelopmental hypothesis of schizophrenia: following a trail of evidence from cradle to grave. Developmental Psychopathology. 12:501-527.

McGee, R., Silva, P.A., and Williams, S. P. (1984). Perinatal, neurological, environmental and developmental characteristics of seven-year-old children with stable behaviour problems. Journal of Child Psychology and Psychiatry, 25, 573-586.

Mednick, S.A., Kandel, E. (1988). Genetic and perinatal factors in violence. In: S.A. Mednick, T. Moffitt, (Ed). Biological Contributions to Crime Causation (pp. 331). Dordrecht: Martinus Nijhoff.

Murray RM, Jones PB, Susser E, Van Os J and Cannon M. (2003). The Epidemiology of Schizophrenia. Cambridge University Press, New York, N.Y.

Neugebauer R. (2005). Accumulating evidence for prenatal nutritional origins of mental disorders. JAMA.294, 621-623.

Neugebauer, R.N., Hoek, H.W., Susser, E. (1999). Prenatal exposure to wartime famine and development of antisocial personality disorder in early adulthood. Journal of the American Medical Association, 282, 455-462.

Neugebauer R. (1997). The uses of psychosocial epidemiology in promoting refugee health. American Journal of Public Health, 87, 726-728.

Olds, D., Henderson, C.R. Jr, Cole, R., et al. (1998). Long-term effects of nurse home visitation on children's criminal and antisocial behavior: 15-year follow-up of a randomized controlled trial. Journal of the American Medical Association, 280, 1238-1244.

Paulhus, D.L., Martin, C.L. (1986). Predicting adult temperament from minor physical anomalies. Journal of Personality and Social Psychology, 50, 1235-1239.

Pine, D.S., Cohen, P., Brook, J., and Coplan, J.D. (1997). Psychiatric symptoms in adolescence as predictors of obesity in early childhood. American Journal of Public Health, 87, 1303-1310.

Raine, A., Brennan, P., Mednick, S.A. (1994). Birth complications combined with early maternal rejection at age 1 year predispose to violent crime at age 18 years. Archives of General Psychiatry, 51, 984-988.

Raine, A. (1993). The Psychopathology of Crime: Criminal Behavior as a Clinical Disorder. San Diego: Academic Press.

Ravelli, G.P., Stein, Z.A., Susser, M.W. (1976). Obesity in young men after famine exposure in utero and early infancy. New England Journal of Medicine. 295, 349-353.

Ravelli, A.C., van der Meulen, J.H., Michels, R.P., et al. (1998). Glucose tolerance in adults after prenatal exposure to famine. Lancet., 351,173-177.

Reiss, A.J. and Roth, J.A. (Eds.). (1993). Understanding and Preventing Violence, Vol. 1. Washington, DC: National Academy Press.

Robinson, N.M. and Robinson, H.B.(1965) A follow-up study of children of low birth weight and control children at school. Pediatrics. ,35:425-433.

Roseboom, T.J., van der Meulen, J.H., Ravelli, A.C., Osmond, C., Barker, D.J., Bleker, O.P. (2001). Effects of prenatal exposure to the Dutch famine on adult disease in later life: an overview. Twin Research. Rothman, K.J. and Greenland, S. (1998). Modern Epidemiology. (2nd ed.), Philadelphia: Lippincott-Raven Publishers.

St. Clair D, Zu M, Wang P, Yu Y, Fang Y, Zhang F, Zheng X, Gu N, Feng G, Sham P and He L. (2005). Rates of adult schizophrenia following prenatal exposure to the Chinese Famine of 1959-1961. JAMA 294, 557-62. Sampson, R.J., Raudenbush, S.W., Earls, F. (1997). Neighborhoods and violent crime: a multilevel study of collective efficacy. Science. 277, 918-924. Stein, Z., Susser, M., Saenger, G., Marolla, F. (1975). Famine and Human Development The Dutch Hunger Winter of 1944-45. New York: Oxford University Press. Stein, Z., Susser, M., Saenger, G., Marolla, F. (1973). Nutrition and mental performance. Science. 178(62), 708-713.

Suomi S.J. (1997). Long-term effects of different early rearing experiences on social, emotional and pyshiological development in nonhuman primates. In: Neurodevelopement and Adult Psychopathology. Ch. 8, Keshavan MS, Murray RM, eds, Cambridge, UK: Cambridge University Press, pp. 104-116.

Susser, E., Hoek, H.W., Brown, A. (1998). Neurodevelopmental disorders after prenatal famine: The story of the Dutch Famine Study. American Journal of Epidemiology. 147, 213-216.

Susser, E. and Lin, S.P. (1992). Schizophrenia after prenatal exposure to the Dutch Hunger Winter of 1944-45. Archives of General Psychiatry. 49, 983-988.

Susser, E., Neugebauer, R., Hoek, H.W., et al. (1996). Schizophrenia after prenatal famine: Further evidence. Archives of General Psychiatry. 53, 25-31.

Terry, M.B. and Susser, E. (2001). Commentary: The impact of fetal and infant exposures along the life course. International Journal of Epidemiology. 30, 95-96.

Van Os J, Selten J-P (1998). Prenatal exposure to maternal stress and later schizophrenia: the May 1940 invasion of the Nehterlands. British Journal of Psychiatry 172, 324-326.

Waldrop, M.F., Bell, R.Q., McLaughlin, B. and Halverson, C.F. (1978). Newborn minor physical anomalies predict short attention span, peer aggression, and impulsivity at age 3. Science, 199, 536-565.

World Health Organization. (1948). Manual of the International Classification of Diseases, Injuries and Causes of Death, (6th ed). Geneva: World Health Organization. World Health Organization. (1938). Manual of the International Statistical Classification of Diseases, Injuries, and Causes of Death. Geneva: World Health Organization. Zeldenrust ELK. (1966) Psychopathie. Ned Tijdschr Geneeskd. 110:1737-1745.

Index

A

B

C

D

E

F

G

H

I

J

K

L

M

N

O

P

Q

R

T

U

V

W

Y